WORKING WITH
DYSPRAXICS

A PRACTICAL GUIDE TO THERAPY FOR DYSPRAXIA

WORKING WITH
DYSPRAXICS

A PRACTICAL GUIDE TO THERAPY FOR DYSPRAXIA

SUSAN HUSKINS MSc MCST

Series Editor: Gill C Darvill

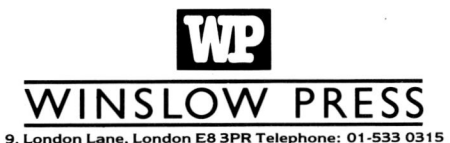

WINSLOW PRESS

9, London Lane, London E8 3PR Telephone: 01-533 0315

First published in 1986 by Winslow Press,
9 London Lane, London E8 3PR

ISBN 0 86388 040 1

J5148/DESIGN + PRINT/REDESIGN PRINT/01-533 2631

CONTENTS

CHAPTER 1
INTRODUCTION
1

CHAPTER 2
DIFFERENTIAL
DIAGNOSIS
– NON VERBAL FORMS
7

CHAPTER 3
DIFFERENTIAL
DIAGNOSIS
– APRAXIA OF SPEECH
15

CHAPTER 4
GENERAL PRINCIPLES
OF TREATMENT
29

CHAPTER 5
METHODS OF
TREATMENT
39

CHAPTER 6
TREATMENT:
APPLICATION OF
TECHNIQUES
55

CHAPTER 7
TERMINATING
TREATMENT
73

APPENDIX I
HUSKINS NON-VERBAL
APRAXIA SCREENING
TEST
77

APPENDIX II
DIAGNOSTIC CHECK
LISTS
81

APPENDIX III
ARTICULATORY
DIAGRAMS
88

APPENDIX IV
PROSODIC AND
ARTICULATORY DRILLS
97

BIBLIOGRAPHY
109

GLOSSARY
111

Susan Huskins MSc, LCST

Susan Huskins (née Shorland) qualified as a speech therapist at the West End Hospital Speech Therapy Training School (now part of the National Hospitals College of Speech Sciences) in 1969. She left her first post at the West Middlesex Hospital in Isleworth after three years to study full-time for an MSc in Human Communication Studies which she obtained from Guy's Hospital Medical School in 1974.

After working at Ashford Hospital, Middlesex, she was third-year tutor in the School of Speech Therapy at Birmingham Polytechnic from September 1974 until December 1977. During this period she participated in writing a CNAA degree course, became a College Adviser on Aphasia and related disorders, and published a paper on dysarthria with Dr Pam Grunwell. Her interest in dyspraxia continued throughout this period and in her clinical work with her students she was able to concentrate on adult neurological problems.

Since the birth of two children she has presented a paper on planning treatment for dyspraxic adults and has written on the treatment of articulatory dyspraxia in aphasic patients.

_____**EDITOR'S NOTE**_____

For the sake of clarity alone, in this text we have used 'he' to refer to the patient and 'she' to refer to the therapist.

PREFACE

While theoretical discussions rage about the very existence of articulatory dyspraxia, practising speech therapists are diagnosing it daily in their patients and doing their best to treat this controversial disorder. Many clinicians are working without the benefit of full neurological assessments, CT scans or other sophisticated and 'hi-tech' aids to diagnosis. Many are also working with a highly varied case load of adults and children with the whole range of disorders of voice, speech and language, and are inevitably aware of a lack of specific expertise if they see few dyspraxic patients on a regular basis.

The aim of this book is to draw together current findings on apraxia of speech in adults and to present a meaningful approach to its assessment, diagnosis and treatment. I lay no claim to being originator of the techniques to be discussed but have drawn on examples and methods suggested in the literature over the years, some of which I have used myself in clinical work and some of which have been recommended by experienced colleagues.

It is apparent that much work still needs to be done on refining our diagnostic criteria and rationale of therapy. Also, few studies have been carried out on the efficacy of the treatment techniques to be described. Such studies are necessary if our therapeutic practices are to have proven scientific validity; but as in the field of medicine, the waiting room is full of patients crying out for help now. We, as practicing clinicians, have to offer what help we can on the basis of clinical efficacy – doing what seems to help the patient.

I hope that the reader will resist the temptation to turn straight to the chapter on treatment techniques, but will first spend a little time considering those on assessment and differential diagnosis. References for further reading will be found throughout the text and are summarized in the Bibliography. The Appendices include a screening test, articulatory diagrams and additional articulatory drills. Also, following the Appendices at the end of this book there is a Glossary for those who may be unfamiliar with some of the terms used.

Whilst this book has been in the process of creation, other texts on apraxia in adults have appeared on the market. I have endeavoured to keep the bias of this book practical rather than theoretical and I hope that this 'manual' will fill a gap in our clinical literature and prove a useful everyday guide for speech therapists working with dyspraxic adults.

ACKNOWLEDGEMENTS

I welcome this opportunity to acknowledge the help of many colleagues. My thanks go to John Cameron whose original artwork for my articulatory diagrams meant that many patients had the benefit of clearly presented visual aids. I thank Chris Code for sending a valued pre print and offering the support of looking out for useful references. I also thank Dr Pam Grunwell with whom I worked at Birmingham Polytechnic in the late 1970s for her phonetic and linguistic enlightenment, Judith Langley for her helpful advice, and Gill Darvill for her editorial guidance. In addition I should like to thank those speech therapists working in South Derbyshire who have given valuable support by allowing me access to their case files, clinics and experiences: in particular, Pam Bauer who arranged for me to see interesting patients, Helen Eardley who let me rifle her filing cabinet and Di Pike whose reports of her experiences using Makaton were much appreciated. Finally I must acknowledge the help of my husband John in teaching me to use a word processor and coming to my aid when the system broke down!

CHAPTER 1
INTRODUCTION

Defining the problem /2
Approaching the solution /3
    (a) Identifying different forms of
        apraxia /3
    (b) The importance of differential
        diagnosis /3
    (c) Treatment approaches /5

Chapter 1
INTRODUCTION

Defining the problem

Defining articulatory dyspraxia or apraxia of speech (these terms will be used interchangeably throughout the text), has been problematical since Broca first mentioned Aphemia in 1861 (Brain, 1965). Almost every expert since has renamed the condition and often redefined it, usually in the context of coexisting dysphasia, eg. Luria's afferent and efferent motor aphasia and Schuell's aphasia with sensorimotor impairment and aphasia with persisting dysfluency. However the concept of apraxia of speech as a discrete motor speech disorder was put forward by Darley, Aronson and Brown (1975) and since then the description of this disorder has been subject to scrutiny and clarified as a result. Further research is continually redefining what we know of the physiological basis of this disorder, its motor characteristics and phonetic realisations, in addition to its relationship with dysphasia (with which it frequently co-exists). A review of some of this research is given by Rosenbek, McNeil and Aronson (1984).

This process of redefinition is a reflection of the inevitable evolution of thought on the subject, a process which has accelerated rapidly in recent years with the availability of new techniques for studying the brain and its pathology, such as CT and NMR scans. Advanced technology has also enabled researchers to observe and measure the movements of the articulators more precisely than ever before (Rosenbek et al, 1984). In addition, linguists and phoneticians are becoming more aware of the need for detailed impressionistic phonetic transcription (Grunwell, 1982), as opposed to broad phonemic transcription, if transcriptions of the patient's speech are to be of value both in research and for differential diagnosis. Many studies up to this time, though excellent in other ways, have been ambivalent in their findings because the data used was incomplete, ie. transcribed phonemically rather than phonetically. Without precise tools to measure and record data, even sophisticated analytical and statistical techniques will give, at best, equivocal and, at worst, meaningless results.

The concept of apraxia was originally, and still is, a broad one and includes a variety of movement disorders where there is no paralysis, sensory loss or loss of comprehension of what is required. Brain (1965) put forward a modern definition of apraxia which is still an extremely useful one and can be applied to apraxias affecting limb and facial movements as well as movements of the articulators in speech (articulatory dyspraxia):

> '. . . it is better to think of purposive movement as organised in terms of schemas than in terms of kinaesthetic, motor, visual or other sensory images, a schema being a spatio-temporal disposition which may or may not enter consciousness or may sometimes be conscious and at other times unconscious.
>
> 'Apraxia can then be regarded as a disorganisation of the schemas underlying purposive movement, and ranging from a disturbance at

the highest level, where the schemas are concerned with the formulation of the idea of the movement, down to the lowest level at which the schema consists of a motor pattern which regulates the selection of the appropriate muscles.' Therefore, '. . . apraxia is essentially a disorganisation of the sequence of events in the nervous system in time'.

Rosenbek, Kent and LaPointe discuss this and other models of apraxia in some detail, specifically with regard to apraxia of speech, in the introductory chapter of *Apraxia of Speech: Physiology, Acoustics, Linguistics, Management* (Rosenbek et al, 1984).

Approaching the solution

The relevance of this general definition to practising speech therapists is that some of the adult patients encountered, following CVA or other cerebral trauma, will have an apraxia not necessarily of speech but nevertheless possibly affecting some other aspect of communicative ability, including the patient's performance on aphasia and other tests.

(a) Identifying different forms of apraxia

Bucco-facial (or oral) and ideomotor (or limb) apraxia are two forms of apraxia which will be described in Chapter 2 and which are often found in the more severely affected patient. These disorders may occur in aphasic patients who do not have apraxia of speech, and their presence can initially cause confusion for the therapist making a speech diagnosis. However, some patients present with one or both of these disorders in addition to articulatory dyspraxia and a degree of dysphasia. The picture can be very varied and complex but fortunately not impossible to decipher.

Many, if not most, of the patients encountered by working clinicians have a degree of dysphasia accompanying their articulatory dyspraxia, even if this is only in the early stages of post cerebral trauma. There are comparatively few examples of isolated apraxia of speech. Some patients are severely aphasic with mild articulatory involvement, others mildly dysphasic with severe articulatory difficulties; and yet others have similar degrees of severity of both dysphasia and dyspraxia. All such patients are frequently labelled Broca's aphasics.

Articulatory dyspraxia is generally suspected when the patient is audibly and visibly groping for the correct articulatory postures, when he is dysfluent at an articulatory level (rather than purely because of word finding difficulty); when speech is slow and laboured and full of variable phonetic errors; and when there is obvious difficulty as articulatory complexity increases, with frequent sequencing and substitution errors. Usually the patient's spoken output is far more impaired than one would expect from performance on comprehension, lexic and graphic tasks, though a degree of caution is needed here as both degree of dysphasia present and previous educational level can obviously affect performance in written modalites (reading and writing). The patient is generally aware of his errors and, unlike the fluent (Wernicke's type) dysphasic, makes frequent attempts at self correction. Recent research has added a great deal of detail to the description of apraxia of speech and further consideration will be given to these findings in chapter three.

(b) The importance of differential diagnosis

All clinicians are aware of the need to make an accurate differential diagnosis so that an appropriate treatment regime can be instigated. The problem facing the speech therapist working with adult brain-damaged patients (be it CVA, trauma or other cause of brain damage) is initially to decide what type of communication disorder, if any, the patient has. He may be dysarthric, dysphasic or dyspraxic or even (as with a head injury following RTA) any combination of these. He may have problems with hearing or vision, or be generally confused as is often found in the very elderly CVA patient. He may also be hemiplegic and he may have a bucco-facial or a limb apraxia in addition to his other difficulties.

Having established, using appropriate assessments such as the MTDDA, the BDAE or the PICA, whether or not he is dysphasic, the clinician must then determine if he also has articulatory problems and whether these are dysarthric or dyspraxic in nature.

The differential diagnosis between fluent dysphasic errors (literal paraphasias) and errors due to articulatory dyspraxia, has caused much confusion in the past. Detailed guidelines will be presented in Chapter 3. The presence of bucco-facial or oral apraxia in some patients has only served to increase this confusion. There has been far less difficulty recognising dysarthric problems when they are present. Paradoxically, it is often easier to diagnose severe articulatory dyspraxia than milder forms, where speech errors can be confused initially with the literal paraphasias of dysphasia. However, differentiating between bucco-facial and articulatory apraxia (ie the most severe forms of these disorders) may be a problem, and such conditions may be confused with aphasia or anarthria by the less experienced clinician. They may of course coexist with a variable degree of dysphasia.

The treatment strategies for dysphasia are inevitably quite different from those for dyspraxia and dysarthria, even though the broader management issues may overlap considerably. Dysphasia is a disorder of language, hence the rationale of treatment is aimed at improving language performance in all modalities (auditory, lexic, oral and graphic, ie. heard, read, spoken and written language). In dysarthria, language is intact and only speech production impaired; but in many cases, several of the speech mechanisms are involved necessitating attention to respiratory, phonatory, resonatory and articulatory performance (ie. breathing, voice, nasality and speech) as appropriate.

The rationale for the treatment of dyspraxia is even more complex since there are still arguments about the fundamental nature of the disorder. Both Luria and Schuell have regarded the more severe forms (afferent motor aphasia and aphasia with sensorimotor impairment respectively) as a sensorimotor articulation disorder occurring with dysphasia. This school of thought has given rise to treatment techniques which emphasise both sensory stimulation (tactile and auditory), and motor exercises in the context of appropriate language therapy.

More recently, the work of Darley and many others has emphasised that apraxia of speech is a motor speech disorder and some research results appear to substantiate this, particularly in patients with moderate or mild disorder (Rosenbek et al, 1984). Hence the emphasis in recent literature is on treating the patient's articulation difficulties in a very direct way, working on articulatory sequencing, consonant clusters and polysyllabic words etc. Rosenbek does recognise, however, that many dyspraxic patients are also dysphasic to a degree, often early in their recovery.

It is tempting to conclude that Schuell and Luria were describing much more severely impaired patients than those encountered by Darley and Rosenbek. This view is substantiated by the fact that both Schuell and Luria including a less severe category of dyspraxic patients (Shuell's aphasia with persisting dysfluency and Luria's efferent motor dysphasia). The treatment techniques they suggest for these groups of patients have far more in common with Darley and Rosenbek's ideas than the severe categories mentioned earlier. It will be evident from the preceding discussion, that the degree of severity of the patient's disorder is of considerable importance when planning treatment. The severely apraxic patient needs articulation work at a much more basic level than one who is mildly or moderately impaired. The severity of any accompanying dysphasia is bound to influence the way in which speech work can be approached and, in addition, has considerable bearing on the prognosis as both Rosenbek (1984) and Wertz (1984) point out. No two patients are exactly alike and no two have exactly the same profile of dysphasic and dyspraxic difficulties. This means that assessment must be thorough, and treatment individually tailored, even if some of the treatment is ultimately carried out in a group situation.

(c) Treatment approaches

In order to simplify this complex area, treatment strategies and tactics will be considered in relation to different levels of severity of the dyspraxia and any coexisting dysphasia. Such divisions are quite arbitrary but are felt to be clinically justified and hence a useful way of presenting ideas for treatment. Apart from Wertz (1984), recent literature has given few guidelines for coping with the most severely affected patients. An attempt will therefore be made, in Chapters 4, 5, and 6 to review possible approaches to their management, including the use of alternative methods of communication. A variety of techniques to help the severely and moderately impaired dyspraxic patient will be discussed including the use of articulatory diagrams, reauditorization and prosodic approaches. No pretence is made of offering new revelations or innovations in treatment. The treatment methods to be discussed are by and large those tried and tested by expert clinicians here and abroad over many years. These can now be combined with newer and more experimental approaches (such as the use of a pacing board); and their rationales are also mentioned where appropriate. Finally, those patients with mild and minimal articulatory dyspraxia will be considered and various treatment programmes and drills will be reviewed.

Given that there is still ambiguity about the exact nature of articulatory dyspraxia and a great deal of experimental work is still going on, it is impossible to be dogmatic about treatment. An eclectic approach has served well in the past and must continue to do so. In this way, traditional methods may be combined with new and more experimental approaches to provide the maximum possible benefit for any individual patient. Prior to this discussion of current techniques in Chapters 5 and 6, consideration will be given in Chapter 4, to more general strategies and management issues which are equally important when working with dyspraxics.

CHAPTER 2
DIFFERENTIAL DIAGNOSIS
– NON VERBAL FORMS

Different forms of dyspraxia /8
    (a) Ideomotor apraxia /8
    (b) Buccofacial (and oral) apraxia /10
    (c) Constructional apraxia /10
Limitations of standardised assessment procedures /11
A screening test for non-verbal apraxias /12
    (a) The test design /12
    (b) The test format: administration and scoring /12
    (c) Interpretation of the test /13

CHAPTER 2
DIFFERENTIAL DIAGNOSIS
– NON VERBAL FORMS

Different forms of dyspraxia

The speech therapist is likely to meet other forms of dyspraxia apart from apraxia of speech. Some of these may affect a patient's performance on assessment tasks, obscure the differential diagnosis in other ways or even affect the mode of therapy. Most commonly encountered in the average hospital caseload are ideomotor (limb) apraxia, buccofacial (including oral) apraxia and sometimes, constructional apraxia. These are described below because they do occur in some dysphasic patients – generally the more severely affected – and they can present a puzzling picture for the clinician.

(a) Ideomotor apraxia

An ideomotor apraxia of the unparalysed (left) hand has been reported many times in patients with a right hemiplegia and aphasia. (Brain, 1965; Geschwind, 1965; Luria, 1970). Whether this is a 'true' apraxia, or the result of a callosal disconnexion syndrome, is not an issue to be debated here. Such patients may be unable to copy movements with the left (apraxic) hand even though it is not paralysed (Brain, 1965; Head, 1963; Travis, 1972). The patient with ideomotor apraxia may be able to manipulate objects quite adequately with the affected hand (eg. use a comb, toothbrush or pencil correctly) but be unable to mime or imitate the gesture involved. This inability to use gesture with the unparalysed arm has obvious implications for the severely speech impaired patient, since it dramatically limits the potential for use of gesture or mime for communication. A patient with this type of apraxia is unlikely to master a sign system such as Amerind or Makaton unless the ideomotor apraxia resolves or is amenable to treatment. Another and more subtle problem is that the patient's ability to point to command may be affected in severe cases. Many of our tests of auditory comprehension involve commands to point to various objects, pictures or body parts. A patient with ideomotor apraxia may perform badly on comprehension tests because of his limb involvement rather than because of failure to comprehend the language used. However, he may be seen to be eye pointing when finger pointing has failed. The assessment of such patients requires skilful observation to ascertain if they do understand verbal commands, in addition to assessment of ideomotor function. A screening test for ideomotor, oral and constructional apraxia can be found in Appendix I; and details of the test and its administration are given later in this chapter. A more detailed screening test for limb apraxia can be found in Code and Gaunt (1986), where pantomime, sybolic gesture, tool use and pantomime sequence are all separately assessed.

An example of ideomotor (limb) apraxia in an aphasic patient was seen in Mrs PS, a 45-year-old lady who had suffered an embolic CVA. She had a dense right hemiplegia so had to use her left hand for the test items. On the screening test (*see Appendix I*) she was frequently unable to carry out commands though her efforts suggested that she had understood what was required. On demonstration (this was the aspect which was scored on most occasions) she typically produced a less than perfect performance, with only one outright incorrect response recorded. Responses were very typical of a degree of limb apraxia in that they were 'on the right lines' but frequently inaccurate in detail such as the precise position of fingers, number of fingers used or use of thumb instead of fingers. Her responses on the ideomotor section of the test can be seen in Table 1 below.

Table 1. Results of Mrs PS on Ideomotor Praxis subtest:

Ideomotor tasks	Score		Comment
	C	D	
make fist		2	
thumbs up		1	eventually
wave goodbye		1	
say /ʃ/		0	used thumbs up
point way out	1	0	used whole hand then thumb. Gesture worse after demonstration
salute		1	slight orientation problem
victory V		1	eventually correct
comb hair		1	patted hair
light match		1	match against chair
seal letter		2	eventually

SCORE TOTAL: 11/20

KEY: C = to command. D = after demonstration

SCORING: 2 = perfect performance
1 = imperfect but acceptable
0 = fail

(b) Buccofacial (and oral) apraxia

This form of apraxia affects the ability to imitate, or to carry out to command, facial and oral movements. Such movements occur quite normally in spontaneous situations (eg. the patient can smile, frown, chew, swallow or whistle in appropriate situations) but these same activities cannot be produced voluntarily (Brain, 1965; Head, 1963).

The occurrence of severe oral apraxia with aphasia was also observed in Mrs PS, mentioned above. Even after repeated demonstrations, her ability to carry out simple oral tasks was extremely limited. She frequently needed help to achieve the desired oral gesture. For example, when attempting to protrude her tongue, she grimaced, opened her mouth wide, moved her tongue around inside her mouth and generally made a great deal of effort without producing the desired result. (This is very typical of apraxics.) Mrs PS realised that she was not producing the correct response so was encouraged to use her left hand to get hold of her tongue. Eventually she managed to pull her tongue to the right position using her fingers. Immediately after this her ability to protrude her tongue voluntarily and to command improved dramatically, demonstrating ability to relearn and improve performance. (Not all apraxics are so competent!) Her responses on the oral praxis subtest of the screening test can be seen in Table 2.

This type of apraxia is often seen in patients with Broca's aphasia but can also be found in patients with Wernicke's aphasia (Ajuriaguerra and Tissot, in Vinken and Bruyn, 1970). In other words, buccofacial, or at least oral, apraxia can be found in patients with severe dysphasia *with* or *without* articulatory dyspraxia. Thus the presence of oral dyspraxia does not necessarily mean that the patient also has articulatory dyspraxia, though this is often the case. There are instances where the patient's speech is quite fluent (though full of 'literal paraphasias' as in Wernicke's aphasia) in spite of the presence of oral apraxia. The less experienced clinician may easily be confused by the presence of oral apraxia; and fluent phonological speech errors (literal paraphasias) may be wrongly attributed to articulatory dyspraxia, in spite of the lack of 'articulatory' difficulty. Treatment strategies may then, incorrectly, include much emphasis on retraining articulatory movements (not necessary for this type of patient) with consequent neglect of auditory training and stimulation which are far more beneficial to the patient with fluent phonological problems and poor self-monitoring.

(c) Constructional apraxia

This is generally associated with right hemisphere damage and hence is encountered far less frequently by speech therapists working with dysphasic adults. The reason it is included here is that, occasionally, a patient's writing may be affected by this type of apraxia (Critchley, 1953, Brain, 1965; Luria, 1970). It is quite obviously not a written language deficit but affects the ability to construct letter shapes, to draw or even to arrange blocks or matchsticks to a given pattern. Attempts at writing (both spontaneous and copying) give rise to overlapping of letters, omissions of parts of letters and otherwise inaccurate reproduction. The patient is frequently unaware of his errors (Brain, 1965). Examples of poor performance on the constructional praxis subtest of the screening test can be seen in *Figure 5*, page 79. For comparison, normal performance on the same subtest can be seen in *Figure 4*, page 78.

Limitations of standardised assessment procedures

The assessment of non-verbal forms of dyspraxia has often been a problem for the speech therapist because most readily available aphasia tests do not cover these disorders. An exception to this is the Boston Diagnostic Aphasia Examination (BDAE) by Goodglass and Kaplan (1972). A particularly useful section in this test is that containing supplementary non-language tests. The items of interest here are the tests for buccofacial, limb and constructional apraxias. More recently, another much more specific test has become available in this country, the Apraxia Battery for Adults by Barbara Dabul (Dabul, 1979). Though this is primarily a test for apraxia of speech, subtest III is specifically designed to diagnose limb apraxia and oral apraxia. There are 10 test items for each type of apraxia in this subtest, and a 6-point scoring system is used.

Table 2. Results of Mrs PS on Oral Praxis subtest:

Oral tasks	Score C	Score D	Comment
protrude tongue	0	0	only able to do with assistance of hand
smile	1		slight delay
look glum		1	
swallow		1	needed demo of drinking
lick lips		0	moved tongue around inside mouth
whistle		0	eventually pursed lips with help
kiss		1	after much demo
blow out match		0	put match into mouth
smoke cigarette		0	made drinking action
click tongue		0	could not do voluntarily but tutted in frustration

SCORE TOTAL: 4/20

KEY: C = to command. D = after demonstration

SCORING: 2 = perfect performance

                 1 = imperfect but acceptable

                 0 = fail

A screening test for non-verbal apraxias

Not all clinicians have access to the Apraxia Battery for Adults or even the BDAE. For those who do not, the screening test for oral, ideomotor and constructional apraxias provided in Appendix I (page 77) will help in isolating these non-verbal problems.

(a) The test design

The test is designed to be used in conjunction with standardised aphasia tests, as a supplementary procedure. Interpretation of results is obviously affected by the degree and type of concurrent aphasia and any sensory or motor impairment. It was based (like Dabul's subtest III) on one designed by De Renzi, Pieczuro and Vignolo (1966).

This author expanded the above test to include tests for constructional apraxia in addition to bucco-facial (or oral) and ideomotor (limb) apraxia. The basic outline and scoring system devised by De Renzi et al was used, but the test items were modified to incorporate classical tests for apraxia from elsewhere in the literature. In particular the ideomotor section was considerably modified to make the tasks more culturally appropriate and to bring in two items of greater complexity. The tests of constructional praxis sample two-dimensional abilities using pencil and paper and matchstick designs and three-dimensional abilities using match boxes as building blocks. The rationale of the test was based on its grounding in classical theories on the subject of apraxia and the regular use of similar tests of praxic function by workers in the field. A reliability study was carried out by the author on 10 neurologically stable patients, after which the test was found to be adequate for screening purposes. It was then used on 35 patients in a study by the author as part of an MSc project (Huskins, 1973).

(b) The test format: administration and scoring

There are ten items in each part of the test and responses are scored on a three-point scale. A subject scores 0 if his response is incorrect, 1 for a passable but not perfect attempt and 2 for a normal performance. Commands are given both orally and by use of demonstration (since this is not a test of comprehension but of performance); and it is useful to note whether the subject responds to the oral command or only to the demonstration.

The oral tasks do not require the use of objects; but if a patient fails on items 8 and 9 it is interesting to see the response with the real objects (a match and a cigarette respectively). Item 7 involves kissing the hand or blowing a kiss, but only the oral gesture of kissing is scored. For the ideomotor and drawing tasks the patient is always asked to use the left hand even if he is not hemiplegic (assuming that if he is he will have a right hemiplegia). If the patient is not hemiplegic or wishes to use the right hand, it is useful to test both right and left hands separately. Items 9 and 10 on the ideomotor test should be attempted initially *without* real objects, to test higher-level pantomime ability. If the patient fails, the clinician should provide real objects and note what difference this makes to his performance. Difficulty using real objects in a sequence may indicate the presence of ideational problems (ideational apraxia). These are problems at a higher level of organisation than ideomotor apraxia (Brain, 1965). Examples of a typical apraxic patient's performance on these two subtests of the screening test can be seen in Tables 1 and 2.

The tests of constructional praxis require six match boxes, some matches and pencil and paper. Before proceeding it is important to check that the patient's visual perception is adequate for the following tasks. Usually this has been covered in previous testing as in the visual and reading subtests of the Minnesota test. The examiner builds a model using three of the match boxes and asks the patient to copy it using the other three. In the drawing subtest, the examiner draws the simple figures of a circle, triangle, cross and house, or presents such drawings to be copied by the patient. (The original stimulus pictures for this subtest can be found in *Figure 3*, page 78.) In drawing tasks the use of the unaccustomed hand must be taken into account when scoring. Similarly matchstick patterns are made for the patient to copy. This is not a test of memory so that all the models are left out until the patient has copied them. Those without problems will frequently act on the verbal command alone. However the patient with constructional apraxia will have great difficulty making these models in spite of adequate perception. In addition, his writing will show characteristics already described, eg. badly shaped letters, over-writing, etc, as seen in *Figure 5*, page 79.

(c) Interpretation of the test

It must be remembered that this screening test is not a test of comprehension but of the patient's output. It is assumed that any difficulty with comprehension of speech has been covered by prior aphasia assessment. One is not noting the patient's failure to respond to oral commands but his failure to imitate a demonstration. Bearing this in mind, failure on any of these test items indicates the possible presence of that particular form of apraxia; and the lower the patient's score, the more certain the diagnosis. If this screening test is used in conjunction with the usual aphasia test batteries, it should give an additional useful insight into the patient's disorder by allowing the clinician to decide whether the patient has an oral or a limb apraxia, and to what extent this affects his performance on other tests. The presence of bucco-facial or oral apraxia does not necessarily mean that the patient will also have an articulatory dyspraxia, as mentioned earlier. Oral apraxia frequently accompanies fluent (Wernicke's) aphasia but does not itself affect the patient's speech. The presence of ideomotor apraxia is particularly significant in a speechless patient where alternative means of communication are being considered. Where such a limb apraxia exists, the prognosis for learning and using a manual sign system is usually very poor. It is obviously important for this condition to be diagnosed early and monitored regularly in the more severely impaired patients so that tests of comprehension can be properly interpreted and decisions made about the value, if any, of teaching alternative methods of communication.

DIFFERENTIAL DIAGNOSIS – APRAXIA OF SPEECH

Making the diagnosis /16
Articulatory dyspraxia: phonetic or phonological disorder /16
    (a) Method of transcription /16
    (b) Classification of patients /17
Characteristics of articulatory dyspraxia /18
    (a) First impressions /18
    (b) Rosenbek's description /18
    (c) Phonetic characteristics /19
    (d) Wertz's description/20
Limitations of standardised assessment procedures – apraxia of speech /20
    (a) Aphasia tests /20
    (b) Tests for apraxia of speech /21
    (c) Interpretation of data/22
Diagnostic check lists /22
    (a) Origins of the check lists /22
    (b) Features of dysarthria /23
    (c) Features of dysphasia /23
    (d) Features of dyspraxia /23
    (e) Suggestions for scoring/27
Looking forward/27

CHAPTER 3
DIFFERENTIAL DIAGNOSIS
– APRAXIA OF SPEECH

Making the diagnosis

One cannot actually diagnose articulatory dyspraxia unless the patient is able to produce some speech for analysis. In spite of this, clinicians do quite confidently make such a diagnosis, even in speechless patients, though Wertz et al (1984) advise a 'wait and see' approach. The criteria for diagnosis in these very severe cases seems to be the absence of speech in the presence of moderate to good language performance on aphasia tests, and the absence of any neuromuscular impairment of an anarthric nature. Such a patient can spontaneously chew, swallow, cough and smile quite normally, but is unable even to phonate voluntarily. He is also quite unable to imitate speech, read aloud or name pictures; and any attempts to speak produce characteristic groping articulatory postures. There is great hesitation, and the patient may inhibit responses which he senses are obviously going to turn out wrong. In contrast, some patients who display some of the obvious characteristics of oral apraxia, have remarkably well preserved automatic speech and may swear fluently and clearly, though spontaneous speech is virtually absent. Aphasia tests should identify whether this latter group of patients is in fact predominantly aphasic with an oral apraxia, or suffering from apraxia of speech. Another group of speechless patients has no such automatic speech, but is handicapped by a recurrent utterance or by perseveration on a word or syllable. Oral apraxia is often present as before, and these patients are usually severely dysphasic. As patients in these last two groups recover, they may well be found to have some degree of apraxia of speech.

The diagnostic criteria put forward by Darley (1975), and later by Rosenbek (1984), are difficult if not impossible to apply to these very severe cases but are of much greater value in diagnosing moderately impaired patients. The same is true of the phonetic and phonological techniques suggested by Grunwell (1982), which are of great value in differentiating the articulatory (phonetic) errors of dyspraxia from the literal paraphasias (phonological errors) of dysphasia.

Articulatory dyspraxia: phonetic or phonological disorder

(a) Method of transcription

One reason why arguments about the nature of articulatory dyspraxia have continued to abound in the literature, is that different researchers have collected data in different ways, many of them using a broad phonemic transcription which can conceal almost as much as it reveals about the patient's speech. (Wertz et al, 1984, also make this point). An example of the difficulties created by this approach is given by Ruth Lesser (1978) in her analysis of Blumstein's work on the phonological problems of dysphasics (including dyspraxic ones). She describes how Blumstein appears to have used a broad rather than a narrow phonetic transcription and comments:

'It appears to be at this higher level of phonological encoding rather than at the phonetic level that all aphasias show the same quality; a narrow phonetic transcription would presumably have distinguished the Broca's aphasics with laboured speech and impaired articulatory agility from the other two groups.' (ie. Wernicke's and Conduction aphasics).

Lesser goes on to discuss many of the recent studies of dysphasic and dyspraxic speech in far more detail than can be summarised here; but it is clear that until all researchers transcribe their data in the same way, comparison of their results will not be very enlightening.

(b) Classification of patients

Another fundamental problem with many of these studies is the way in which the patients are classified clinically. Catherine MacKenzie (1982) observes that two distinctive patterns of impairment were seen in her aphasic subjects: aphasic articulatory defect and aphasic phonological defect. She points out that Darley's apraxia of speech category 'encompasses both types of subject', and observes that 'the term 'apraxia' has been over-applied and misapplied' to such an extent that it is no longer a useful label. So it seems that the very categories of patients we use, or the way we classify them, needs to be made more specific; and this can only be done if our data is collected and recorded using more refined and accurate techniques, including more precise phonetic transcription.

However, accurate phonetics is not the only solution to the problem. Rosenbek (1984) discusses how our ears can deceive us so that we perceive speech errors as phonemic when acoustic analysis reveals a more complex articulatory distortion. Duffy and Gawle's paper (1984) expands this argument. Unfortunately, most clinicians do not have access to suitable instrumentation to supplement their auditory perception of the patient's speech. However Rosenbek points out how important it is to train clinicians to use narrow phonetic transcription of speech when instrumentation is not available, and he notes, as Lesser did, how infrequently such transcription has been used in past studies of apraxia of speech.

It is not surprising then that patients classified as having apraxia of speech are frequently found on closer scrutiny to be both dysphasic and dyspraxic with both dysphasic phonological impairment and articulatory (phonetic) problems overlapping. Itoh and Sasanuma (1984) discuss the difficulty of finding a patient with an isolated articulatory dyspraxia for study, and reiterate the point that Darley's description of apraxia of speech encompasses both phonetic and phonological errors (ie. linguistic as well as motor programming problems).

The clinician working with brain-damaged adults knows that the vast majority of dyspraxic patients also show a degree of dysphasia at some point in their recovery and that the disorders overlap and inevitably impinge on each other. She is also aware that the distinction between dysphasia and apraxia of speech is not solely an academic one, since a different emphasis is required in the treatment of these conditions. A differential diagnosis needs to be made to determine the patient's profile, to establish which condition predominates, and to plan an appropriate treatment programme encompassing all the patient's difficulties. Grunwell (1982) describes how the principles of clinical phonology can be used to help the clinician tease out the phonetic from the phonological errors in the patient's speech. These principles are incorporated in the diagnostic check lists provided later in this chapter.

Characteristics of articulatory dyspraxia

(a) First impressions

Where a patient has some speech, the clinician may get an initial impression of articulatory dyspraxia if he is very dysfluent at an articulatory level and if his speech is effortful, slow and laboured, inaccurate and distorted. He appears to grope for the right starting point and the right sequence of articulatory postures (phonetic experimentation). He is aware of his errors and frequently repeats and self corrects. Further analysis of his speech can be made, preferably from a good tape or video recording or both, to confirm the diagnosis. (NB. a high quality tape recorder is essential to provide clear samples of speech for analysis. Video sound tracks alone are not really adequate, though it is extremely useful to be able to see as well as hear what the patient is doing.)

(b) Rosenbek's description

Rosenbek (1984) suggests the following characteristics of apraxia of speech (summarised in Figure 1). If the patient has articulatory dyspraxia, it will be found that articulation errors increase with the complexity of the speech task (ie. vowels are easiest, consonant clusters most difficult, and most errors occur on initial consonants and phonemes with a lower frequency of occurrence in the

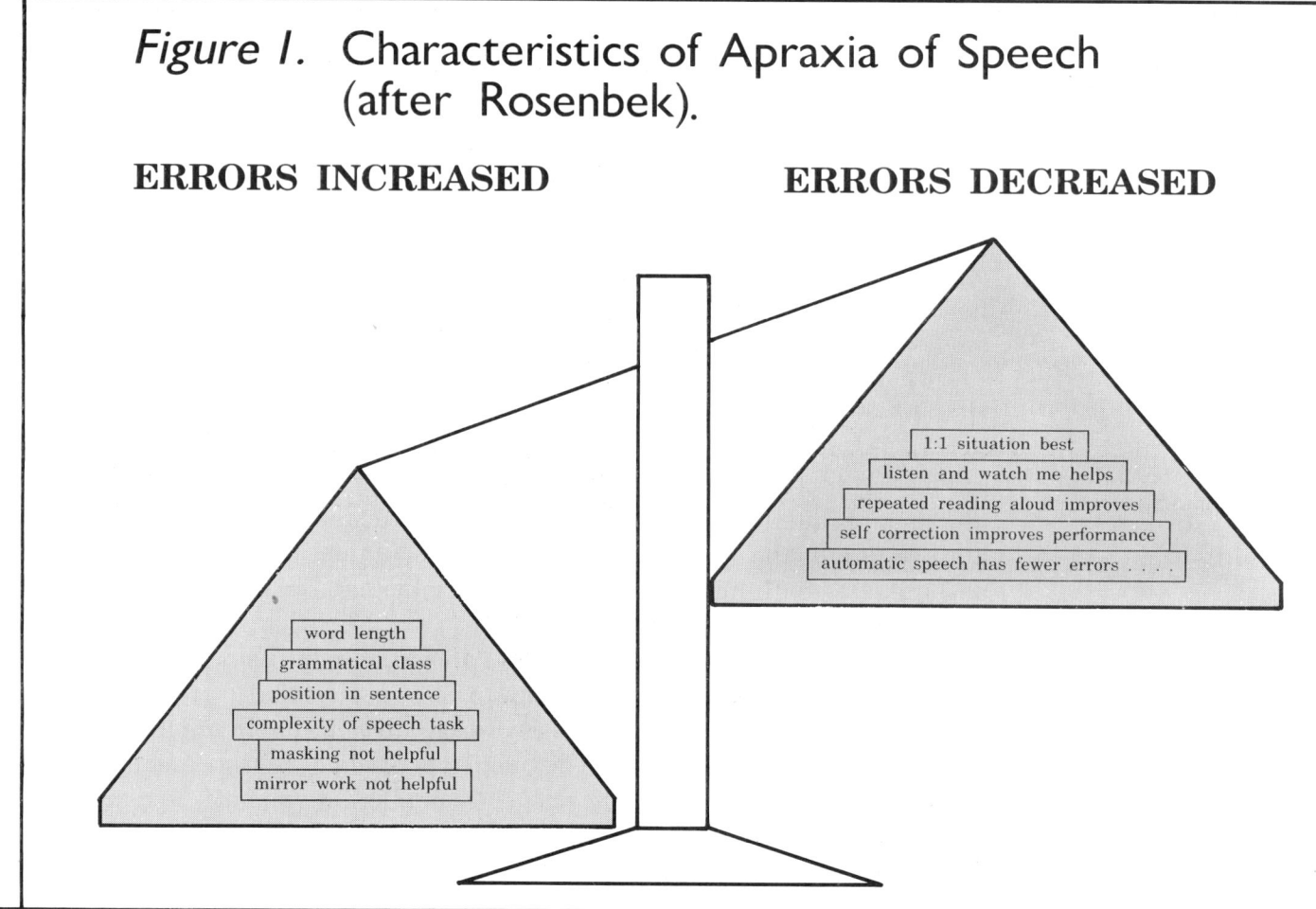

Figure 1. Characteristics of Apraxia of Speech (after Rosenbek).

ERRORS INCREASED

ERRORS DECREASED

1:1 situation best
listen and watch me helps
repeated reading aloud improves
self correction improves performance
automatic speech has fewer errors . . . .

word length
grammatical class
position in sentence
complexity of speech task
masking not helpful
mirror work not helpful

language'). Articulation errors also increase with word length and when the weight of psycho-linguistic factors, such as grammatical class and position in a sentence, are considered. Sequencing errors occur but account for only 10% or less of total errors and most substitution errors involve only one or two features. As noted before, automatic speech tends to be better than volitional speech. Self correction by repeated trials of a word tends to lead to improved performance whereas repeated stimulations do not, and stimulus mode also affects performance with best results in a live one-to-one situation. Repeated reading aloud of the same text tends to produce improved performance but the same parts of the text tend to produce difficulty each time. Of specific interest to the speech therapist is the observation that a 'listen and watch me' approach and a one-to-one situation are often found to be helpful, especially to the more severely affected patient. However Rosenbek has found that other facilitators such as masking, monitoring by mirror, delaying responses prior to imitation, and speaking to a strict rhythm, are not helpful.

(c) Phonetic characteristics

As Grunwell (1982) points out, phonetic analysis of the patient's speech reveals variable phonetic errors including weakening of articulations, vowel errors and idiosyncratic substitution. Phonetic sequencing errors do not always simplify: sometimes more complex patterns of articulation and production of non-English sequences occur (ie. phonetic sequences arise which are outside the rules of English phonology). In addition, sounds are sometimes produced which are outside the English phonetic inventory. There are excellent examples of this phenomenon exhibited by one of the author's patients (Mr D) as described by Grunwell in Chapter 5 of *Clinical Phonology* (Grunwell, 1982).

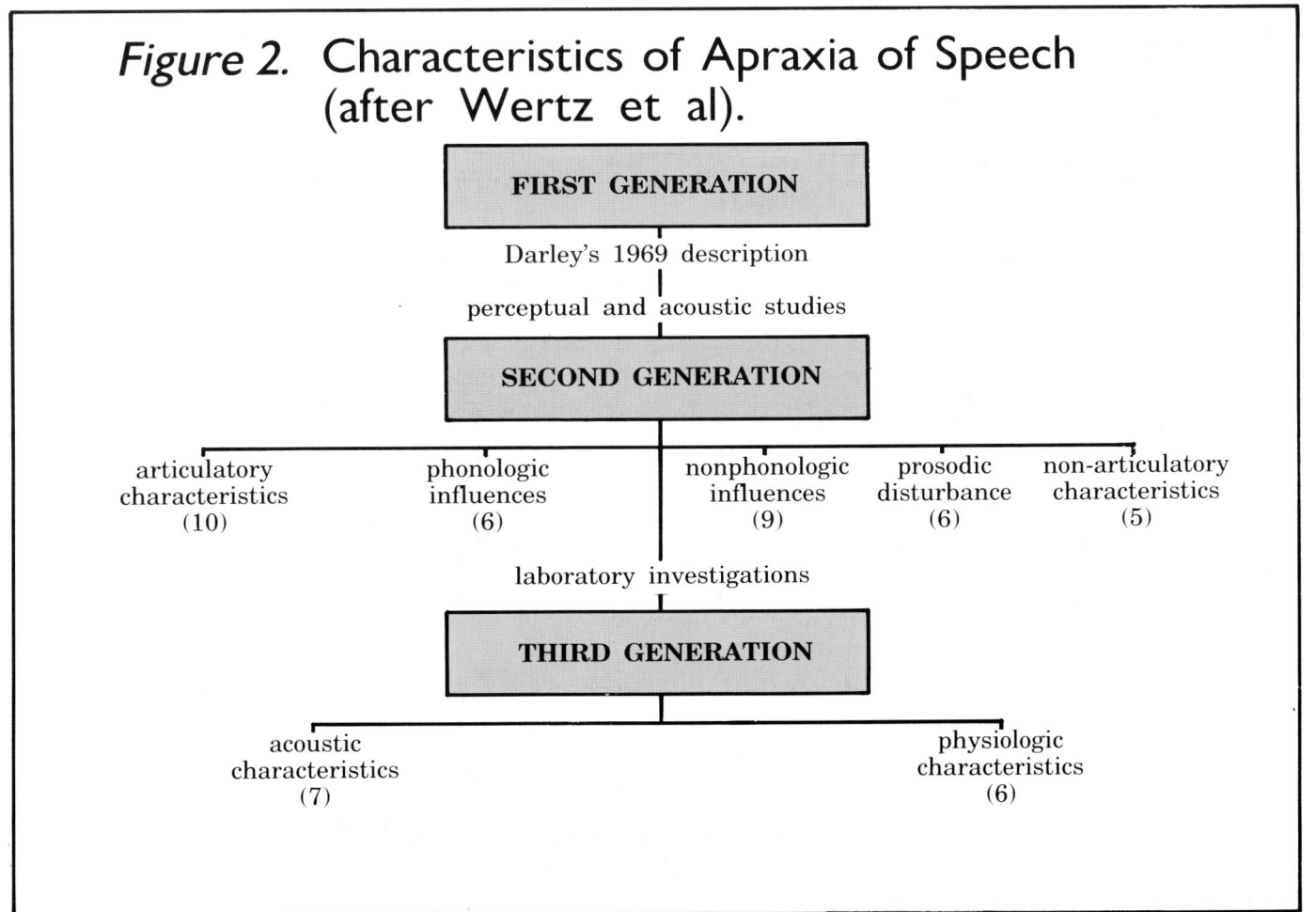

Figure 2. Characteristics of Apraxia of Speech (after Wertz et al).

(d) Wertz's description

Perhaps the fullest description of the characteristics of apraxia of speech is given by Wertz, LaPointe and Rosenbek (1984). This will be summarised below (see also *Figure 2*): Wertz et al review what they call first, second and third-generation characteristics, namely those which have been revised as our knowledge has expanded. The traditional characteristics put forward by Darley in 1969 are described as 'first generation'. The 'second generation', derived from perceptual and acoustic studies, include 10 articulatory characteristics (eg. errors are more likely on consonant clusters than singletons); 6 phonologic influences (eg. accuracy is better for meaningful than non-meaningful utterances); 9 non-phonological influences (eg. watching a mirror has no effect on accuracy of single-word production); 6 aspects of prosodic disturbance (eg. use of inappropriate intersyllabic pauses) and 5 non-articulatory characteristics (eg. there may be a concomitant oral apraxia). Their 'third-generation' characteristics are based on the results of laboratory investigations of the apraxic patient's speech. These include 7 acoustic characteristics (eg. mis-timing of voice onset) and 6 physiologic characteristics (eg. continuous undifferentiated EMG activity).

This very extensive description of apraxia of speech is well worth study, but even the authors themselves condense all the points mentioned into four vital clinical characteristics:

■ Speech is 'effortful with trial-and-error groping articulatory movements and attempts at self-correction'.

■ There is 'dysprosody unrelieved by extended periods of normal rhythm, stress and intonation'.

■ There is 'articulatory inconsistency on repeated productions of the same utterance'.

■ There is 'obvious difficulty initiating utterances'.

Limitations of standardised assessment procedures – apraxia of speech

(a) Aphasia tests

The most commonly used aphasia tests such as the MTDDA, the BDAE and the PICA (Porch Index of Communicative Ability) do not direct the clinician towards a diagnosis of apraxia of speech. However the data collected when carrying out such tests can be utilized to help the clinician arrive at a satisfactory differential diagnosis. The Minnesota Test for the Differential Diagnosis of Aphasia (MTDDA) is based on a theoretical background which was deliberately trying to break away from the early concept of dyspraxia, and therefore does not cover any of the non-verbal forms or refer to articulatory dyspraxia. A diagnosis of 'aphasia with sensorimotor impairment' or the less severe 'aphasia with persisting dysfluency', is the equivalent of a diagnosis of aphasia with apraxia of speech.

Very different in theoretical background is the Boston Diagnostic Aphasia Examination (BDAE). Like the MTDDA, the Boston test does not cover apraxia of speech directly, though as mentioned in Chapter 2, it contains supplementary tests for various non-verbal apraxias. Articulatory dyspraxia is not a concept that exists for Goodglass and Kaplan; though under the heading of pure disorders, they refer to Aphemia (subcortical motor aphasia) which is the equivalent of pure articulatory dyspraxia. The Boston test diagnoses aphasia and, in doing so, classifies aphasics as Broca's, Wernicke's, conduction, transcortical sensory, transcortical motor, global, mixed non-fluent (between Broca's and global) and subcortical. In addition, pure alexia and pure agraphia are described, as is a mixture of the two. The aphasic syndromes of interest here are aphemia and Broca's aphasia.

Some confusion is generated by the fact that Goodglass and Kaplan liken conduction aphasia to Luria's afferent motor aphasia, a syndrome previously associated with the description of combined dysphasia and dyspraxia. This comparison is not particularly clarified when they state that the speech errors in conduction aphasia are literal paraphasias and not articulatory errors, though they admit that 'sometimes the patient's struggle with his literal paraphasias results in an output like that of a Broca's aphasia; and it may be difficult to differentiate the two types of aphasia on the basis of the articulation rating scale'.

The BDAE contains, amongst other things, tests of verbal and non-verbal agility which are very useful, and guidelines for scoring paraphasic errors. The test materials provide a wealth of data but this relies heavily on the clinician's ability to transcribe accurately and interpret results.

(b) Tests for apraxia of speech

In 1979 Barbara Dabul published her Apraxia Battery for Adults in the United States and for the first time a specific test for articulatory dyspraxia became readily available (as mentioned previously, one of the subtests covers oral and limb apraxia). The apraxia battery consists of six subtests measuring diadochokinetic rate, difficulties with increasing word length, presence of oral and limb apraxia, latency and utterance time for polysyllabic words, production on repeated trials and finally, an inventory of 'articulation characteristics of apraxia'. This is an extremely useful test but even so it still does not differentiate clearly between phonetic and phonological errors. As with so many other procedures it is up to the clinician to make this judgement. However it does provide very clear guidelines for observing the other characteristics of apraxia of speech.

In many instances it is found necessary for additional tests and speech tasks to be carried out to confirm the suspected diagnosis of articulatory dyspraxia; and until recently (with the exception of Dabul's Apraxia Battery), clear and systematic guidance was not readily available. However, with the publication of their book *Apraxia of Speech in Adults: The Disorder and its Management*, Wertz, LaPointe and Rosenbek have put forward the most complete approach yet to the appraisal and diagnosis of apraxia of speech (Wertz et al, 1984). They list a whole battery of procedures used on their patients to sample speech and language behaviour and non-verbal intelligence including the PICA, the BDAE, Raven's coloured progressive matrices and the Token Test. Guidance is also given on interpreting the first two tests. Even more valuable is the motor speech evaluation which is described in detail. It is an extremely comprehensive test including repetition of carefully selected sounds, syllables and sequences (eg. p:t:k) and polysyllabic words of increasing articulatory complexity. There is also comparison of mono', di' and polysyllabic words (eg. thick, thicken, thickening), repetition of sentences requiring articulatory dexterity (eg. 'Please put the groceries in the refrigerator'), automatic and volitional counting (up to 20 forwards and backwards), picture description and reading aloud. Methods of collecting and analysing the data are discussed in some detail. In addition, a multi-dimensional scoring system specifically for dyspraxia is included to help determine its severity. Other tests included in the chapter on appraisal and diagnosis are:

■ Tests of isolated oral movements (16 items) eg. 'stick out your tongue'; 'show me your teeth'.

■ Tests of oral motor sequencing (8 items) eg. sequences of two movements such as 'first touch tongue to upper lip, then lower and raise jaw'; and sequences of three movements such as 'click teeth, pucker lips, then lick lips'.

■ Tests to determine the presence of limb apraxia (10 items) eg. 'show me how you wave goodbye'; 'snap your fingers' etc.

(c) Interpretation of data

Assessments such as those described above enable the clinician to collect speech data in a rigorous and systematic way but interpretation of the results still depends on the clinician's knowledge of the characteristics of articulatory dyspraxia as compared with those of the fluent phonological errors (literal paraphasias) of dysphasia. Both types of errors may well appear in the data of dyspraxic patients who are also dysphasic. To make life more difficult, not all clinicians will have access to the procedures described by Wertz et al or Dabul and Bollier; but for those who do not, all is not lost. There are other ways to collect analysable data which can be used to make a differential diagnosis.

Most aphasia assessments include items intended to collect a sample of the patient's speech under different conditions such as imitation, reading aloud and picture description, and including different levels of articulatory and linguistic complexity ranging from repetition of mono' and polysyllabic words (some with consonant blends) through to production of phrases, sentences and continuous speech. Such items are generally scored for overall accuracy and guidelines for more detailed phonetic and linguistic analysis are not normally provided. Some clinicians find it valuable to tape record these test items using a good-quality tape recorder in quiet surroundings, in order to obtain a diverse sample of speech for more detailed analysis. Video tapes of patients performing such test items can give useful additional information. For example, a patient's silent groping for the correct articulatory postures can be seen.

Whilst carrying out an aphasia assessment the clinician is building up an impression of the patient's range of difficulties; and the experienced therapist is usually quickly aware of whether the patient is exhibiting any features of dysarthria or dyspraxia in addition to his dysphasia. For those less experienced in working with brain-damaged adults, a list of the main diagnostic indicators for anarthria, aphasia and apraxia (with and without aphasia) can be found in Table 3, with a similar list for dysphasia and dyspraxia in Table 4 (see pages 24, 25 & 26). The tables are designed to indicate what type of further assessment might be appropriate.

Diagnostic check lists

(a) Origins of the check lists

When a full aphasia assessment has been carried out, and a sample of speech obtained, a provisional analysis of speech behaviour can be carried out with the aid of the diagnostic check lists provided in Appendix I.

These check lists are a modified version of those described at the CST conference at Warwick (Huskins, 1979). They are designed for use with the less severely impaired patient where it is possible to obtain a sample of analysable speech. Though most of the items can be assessed from a tape recording of the patient's speech, some of the items of the dysarthria check list require the presence of the patient and should be dealt with as part of the assessment session. They were originally devised by the author in collaboration with Dr Pam Grunwell at Birmingham Polytechnic in 1977 and were inspired by the work of Darley et al (1972). The author is indebted to Dr Grunwell for the phonetic and linguistic content. The validity of the items in the check lists is substantiated by the recent work of Wertz, Rosenbek and others (see Wertz et al, 1984).

(b) Features of dysarthria

The features of dysarthria are dealt with first. In dysarthria, some or all of the speech mechanisms are impaired together – including respiratory, phonatory, resonatory and articulatory mechanisms. Malfunction in the respiratory mechanism leads to errors of stress, rhythm and rate. Impairment of the phonatory mechanism leads to errors of loudness, intonation and voice quality and even the phonemic voicing feature. When the resonatory mechanism is involved error of oral and nasal resonance, and vowel errors may occur. Where the articulatory mechanism is affected, there may be phonetic errors of manner and place, and articulation rate is frequently abnormal (either too fast or too slow). This speech impairment occurs in the context of neuromuscular weakness of the speech musculature, often with associated bilateral involvement of the limbs. There may be obvious changes in muscle tone (eg spastic or flaccid) and the speech musculature may also exhibit abnormal range and speed of movement. It is not uncommon for those patients who are seriously affected to drool and have swallowing problems, with nasal regurgitation when eating and drinking.

(c) Features of dysphasia

In contrast, the features exhibited by the dysphasic patient are different both neurologically and linguistically. Though he may have a right hemiparesis or hemiplegia and a degree of right facial weakness, his speech musculature and mechanisms are intact. However any speech he produces (the more seriously impaired patients are not included here) may contain semantic, syntactic or morphological errors or a combination of these. He may lack fluency because of a word finding difficulty. Phonological errors also occur but these are the fluent 'substitutions' (eg./tʌp/ for 'cup') and 'transpositions' (eg./pʌk/ for 'cup') of literal paraphasias, namely phonemic errors which obey the rules of English phonology. Substitution errors are usually consonants which differ from the target by only one or two features. Phonemic sequencing errors can also occur including omissions; transpositions (metathesis) such as /hɒdɪleɪ/ for 'holiday'; insertions (especially of vowels) such as /kəlɒk/ for 'clock'; and consonant harmony (a form of perseveration) such as /peɪbl/ for 'table'. Further excellent examples can be found in Grunwell 1982. These phonological errors are frequently reflected in writing as are other linguistic errors. In fact, all language modalities are usually affected to some degree. Auditory comprehension and discrimination may be very poor and impaired auditory monitoring means that the patient does not often self-correct.

(d) Features of dyspraxia

Bearing in mind that the majority of dyspraxic patients also have a degree of dysphasia and may thus exhibit many of the features already described and also that, as Grunwell points out, it is impossible at present to distinguish the neurological source of phonological errors, the final check list aims to highlight those aspects of speech which can be directly attributed to the dyspraxic element of the disorder. While the patient may also present as dysphasic with a right hemiplegia and right facial weakness, a dyspraxic's speech is markedly dysfluent at an articulatory level. Prosody is likely to be disturbed and speech is

Table 3: Main diagnostic indicators

ANARTHRIA

1 Obvious neuromuscular impairment, usually bilateral.

2 Severe feeding difficulties: usually drooling, nasal regurgitation, poor swallowing etc.

3 Comprehension normal.

4 Speech attempts severely distorted by abnormal voice, resonance and articulation.

5 Attempts at gross movements of articulators severely and consistently limited by neuromuscular impairment.

6 If physically capable, may communicate by means of writing or a spelling board.

APHASIA

1 No neuromuscular weakness except possible Right (UMN) facial weakness and Right hemiplegia.

2 No feeding difficulties.

3 Comprehension usually severely impaired.

4 May have some automatic speech.

5 Copies gross movements of the articulators and buccofacial movements. May fail to understand command but can imitate.

6 Reading and writing normally reflect speech and comprehension problems.

APRAXIA

1   No neuromuscular weakness except possible Right (UMN) facial weakness and Right hemiplegia (as aphasia).

2   No feeding difficulties (as aphasia).

3   Comprehension not impaired (unless also dysphasic).

4   Often no speech at all.

5   Frequently cannot copy gross oral movements. May produce wildly aberrant responses demonstrating full range of use of speech musculature.

6   Writing may be affected by constructional apraxia.

APRAXIA WITH APHASIA

1   No neuromuscular weakness except possible Right (UMN) facial weakness and Right hemiplegia (as aphasia and apraxia).

2   No feeding difficulties (as aphasia and apraxia).

3   Comprehension impairment depends on degree of dysphasia.

4   May have no speech or minimal recurrent utterance.

5   Frequently cannot copy gross oral movements. May produce wildly aberrant responses demonstrating full range of use of speech musculature (as apraxia).

6   Frequently unable to write or copy. Communicative ability virtually nil.

Table 4: Main diagnostic indicators

DYSPHASIA

1 Speech may be telegrammatic.
2 Speech may contain free flowing phonemic jargon or phonological errors.
3 Obvious semantic and/or syntactic errors.
4 Comprehension, reading and writing usually affected to some degree.
5 Diadochokinetic rates normal.
6 Variable self monitoring.

DYSPRAXIA

1 Speech halting with disrupted prosody but not truly telegrammatic.
2 Speech dysfluent with articulatory errors.
3 No semantic or syntactic errors unless also dysphasic.
4 No problems with comprehension, reading and writing unless also dysphasic.
5 Diadochokinetic rates usually poor.
6 Self monitoring usually good.

generally slow and laboured. Groping for articulatory postures (phonetic experimentation) can be seen and heard and is a most distinctive feature. Phonetic errors are variable and sometimes idiosyncratic, and speech errors increase with articulatory complexity, ie. consonants are harder than vowels, clusters harder than singletons, and polysyllables harder than monosyllables. Phonetic sequencing errors may occur, but these do not always take the form of simplification. Some phonetic sequences may be produced which do not conform to English phonology; and sometimes sounds are produced which are outside the English phonetic inventory (Grunwell, 1982). However, auditory monitoring may be good, thus leading to frequent and repeated attempts at self-correction. This is particularly true of patients who are primarily dyspraxic rather than dysphasic. There is usually improvement with repeated attempts at words especially where an audio-visual model (listen and watch me) is provided.

(e) Suggestions for scoring

The check lists derived from these observations can be used informally to determine the overall pattern of a patient's disorder with a simple plus or minus scoring system to denote the presence or absence of specific features. A further refinement of the scoring system is to use a rating scale as it gives a more detailed picture of the areas of difficulty. A six-point scale is suggested, where 0 = absence of the feature, 1 = minimal signs, 2 = mild, 3 = moderate, 4 = severe, and 5 = very severe manifestation of a sign or feature. A patient profile can be built up from the check list so that the number of dysarthric, dysphasic and dyspraxic features can be seen at a glance and an average severity rating can be given for each disorder. The more features present for any one disorder, the more certain the diagnosis regardless of severity. This way, an observation that a patient is 'dysphasic but also a bit dyspraxic' may be both qualified and quantified. An example of scoring the check lists and calculating the average severity rating can be found in Appendix II. If the clinician has a large enough sample of transcribable speech (5 to 15 minutes, depending on the rate) and sufficient time to examine the data, a more detailed phonetic and linguistic analysis may be carried out. A good sample of spontaneous speech which can be transcribed orthographically (where targets are known, ie. the sample can be written down longhand because it contains very few completely unintelligible items even though there may be a great many articulatory, phonological, syntactic or semantic errors) is ideal for combined linguistic and phonetic analysis and essential for any research project. It is not essential for the whole of a 15-minute sample to be transcribed phonetically: only those words which are mispronounced would need to be dealt with in such detail.

Looking forward

As Wertz et al (1984) point out, diagnosis is not instantaneous. For severe patients in particular, a period of diagnostic treatment may be necessary to allow for some physiologic recovery and to enable the clinician to explore fully what the patient can and cannot do. This is ultimately as important for making a prognosis and planning treatment as it is for making a differential diagnosis. A salutory observation is also made by the above authors that all these guidelines are based on current knowledge and our existing theoretical framework. Time and further research could well alter our whole perception of the nature of apraxia of speech and, consequently, how to deal with it. However, for the time being, we must act upon what we know.

CHAPTER 4
GENERAL PRINCIPLES
OF TREATMENT

General considerations /30
    (a) Individual versus group treatment /30
    (b) Intensive versus extensive treatment /30
    (c) Integrating speech and language work /31
    (d) Involvement of relatives or nurses /31
    (e) Domiciliary versus hospital therapy /32
    (f) Use of volunteers /32
    (g) Counselling of patient and relatives /33
Evaluation of the prognosis /34
    (a) General pointers /34
    (b) Specific guidelines /35
Alternative methods of communication /35
    (a) Visual systems /36
    (b) New technology /36
    (c) Gestural systems /37
Summary /38

CHAPTER 4
GENERAL PRINCIPLES
OF TREATMENT

General considerations

One of the most important basic principles on which treatment is based is the realistic evaluation of the prognosis for each patient. This is dependent on many factors which will be considered in more detail later. Basically the patient must have adequate health, intelligence and motivation to cooperate with what could well be a lengthy and drawn out treatment. In addition there must be some discernible capacity for relearning. Evaluation of the prognosis is dependent on a full case history and assessment of the patient so that medical and social factors, as well as speech and language ability, are all considered.

Attention will be paid in this section to some of the more general issues raised in the treatment of adult CVA patients with communication problems and how these may affect the person with dyspraxia.

(a) Individual versus group treatment

There is no doubt that dysphasic patients benefit from group treatment, but the patient who also has an articulatory dyspraxia definitely needs to have individual treatment. The direct work needed on articulation is best carried out in a one-to-one situation.

Rosenbek (1984) noted that the speech of dyspraxic patients who only received group treatment where the emphasis was on language work, and who did not receive direct articulation therapy, *did not improve*. This is not to say that dyspraxic dysphasics should be excluded from group work. On the contrary, they should benefit from inclusion in a suitable group ie. one where both articulation and language are given equal consideration, provided that they *also* have ample opportunity for individual work.

(b) Intensive versus extensive treatment

Even in the field of dysphasia, little conclusive research has been carried out on the efficacy of particular methods of treatment. This also applies to the treatment of dyspraxia. It thus seems premature to judge the value of either intensive or extensive treatment until we are much more sure of the methods of treatment we are using. The weight of clinical evidence to date suggests that intensive treatment of any communication problem is preferable to a once-weekly session continuing for months or even years. However, the term 'intensive' means different things to different people: some would regard three one-hour speech therapy sessions per week as intensive. Others would apply the term to two or three sessions per day. In their treatment of dyspraxic patients, Wertz et al (1984) quite clearly fall into the latter group. Their preference is to treat the patient as frequently as possible in the early stages of therapy. How long such a rigorous treatment programme can be maintained appears to be governed as much by how much treatment the patient can afford as by how much stamina he has. In Britain, the majority of patients receiving therapy do so under the National Health Service for which they are not required to pay. However, despite this advantage, there are few centres which can offer such intensive therapy to dyspraxic patients.

For the majority, the choice is limited by what is available. Many British therapists attempt to make up for their inability to provide intensive therapy themselves by involving the patients' relatives as much as possible and by being prepared to offer much more extended therapeutic contact, particularly with the more severely affected patients, over a period of years. Since many eminent clinicians such as Luria, Rosenbek and Schuell have agreed that the treatment of patients with severe dyspraxia can be a very long process but that the patient can continue to make gains over a considerable period of time, such a treatment strategy does seem to have some justification. In most instances, therapists have had to make a practical compromise of maximum regular therapy in the early stages, and long-term follow-up on a regular basis.

(c) Integrating speech and language work

Since so many of these patients are dysphasic *and* dyspraxic, both aspects of their communication problem must be tackled. It is tempting to get carried away by articulation drills, particularly where dyspraxia is the most obvious problem. The kind of approach recommended by Wertz et al (1984) deals very thoroughly with all aspects of work on articulation, but does tend to give the reader the impression that articulation work always comes first. Though this may well be the case with patients who are predominantly dyspraxic, with minimal or no dysphasia, the emphasis must be altered for the average dyspraxic dysphasic. For the latter, Rosenbek (1984) recommends that 'simple articulation training always be but a soupçon of total speech language therapy'.

In Chapter VI, all the examples are of those who are both dysphasic and dyspraxic; and the individual case studies, whilst emphasising therapy for dyspraxia, give some idea of how speech and language work are dovetailed in reality. As a general principle the therapist has to tackle the patient's primary problem most vigorously, be it his dysphasia or his dyspraxia. However, time must be allowed every treatment session for work on his secondary problem. For a patient who is primarily dysphasic with mild dyspraxia, articulation therapy may be covered along with such activities as reading aloud and picture description in addition to drilling selected consonants and blends, or mono' and polysyllabic words, as appropriate.

Where the patient is severely dyspraxic and rather less dysphasic, a large part of each treatment session is likely to be spent in direct speech work, facilitating production of sounds and simple CV, VC or CVC combinations. (It is helpful if the latter are always real words.) These can then be drilled in a language work setting. For example, a therapist wishing to encourage a patient to practise production of the word 'tea' might use the following methods:

■ Closure techniques eg. 'a nice cup of . . . tea'

■ Forced alternatives eg. 'tea or coffee?'

■ Question-and-answer techniques eg. 'what would you like to drink?'.

Such techniques will be described in more detail in Chapter V.

(d) Involvement of relatives or nurses

As mentioned previously, in many British hospitals it becomes imperative to involve relatives and nursing staff in the patient's treatment, since he is likely to derive little benefit from a once-weekly session with the speech therapist in the absence of some back-up. In an ideal world intensive therapy with a fully qualified clinician should be available on a daily basis; but for many this is simply not possible. Therapists often encourage nursing staff and relatives to carry on with treatment started in the clinic. Relatives are frequently invited to sit in on treatment sessions where possible, and where both patient and relative are willing. However, this is only one aspect of their involvement. Since they are an important part of the patient's total communication environment, they need to be counselled on how best to cope with his communication difficulties and how to provide optimum stimulation and support.

For nursing personnel, advice of this nature has to be an ongoing process, since those junior staff in closest daily contact with the patient tend to change frequently. It is essential to form a good working relationship with the senior ward staff (sisters and staff nurses) and ensure that they are kept informed of the patient's speech and language needs and his progress, so that they in turn feel able to instruct their junior staff appropriately. If possible, the speech therapist should arrange to give a general talk on speech and language difficulties to all junior medical ward staff twice or even three times a year, since they move on so frequently to different wards. Particular patients and their speech and language difficulties can be used as examples on such occasions. General principles for helping these patients can be discussed; and an explanation of the speech therapist's role should be provided.

(e) Domiciliary versus hospital therapy

The patient on the ward is easily accessible; and it has been found generally more convenient for the clinician to have patients come to the hospital for outpatient treatment after discharge. Sometimes, however, the benefits of getting out of the house to a stimulating environment can be all but cancelled out by the long wait for ambulance transport at both ends of the day. In addition, it may prove harder to maintain contact with the family when a patient is ferried in for his outpatient appointments.

Domiciliary visits are always helpful, both to assess the home environment and to meet the family. In some instances patients function far better at home than they do in the clinic; and it is always useful to assess functional communication in the most natural setting. It is debatable whether all therapy should, or even could, be carried out on a domiciliary basis but visiting the home on at least one occasion can be an enlightening experience and is to be recommended. An article in the *College of Speech Therapists' Bulletin* (Stevens, 1985) describes domiciliary services for the elderly in Hammersmith and discusses both the value to the patient and the cost effectiveness of such a service.

(f) Use of volunteers

The use of volunteers is becoming quite popular with dysphasic patients, to supplement the often inadequate hospital service. This is not the place to debate whether volunteers can or should substitute for professionally qualified therapists. However, given the very specific problems suffered by dyspraxic patients and the complexity of their problems, they are less likely than those who are simply dysphasic to benefit from the sort of general language stimulation which tends to be provided by volunteers.

The use of a specially trained aide, who observes work with specific patients and carries out specific exercises under the supervision of the clinician, may be more acceptable than the above, particularly where there is a chronic shortage of fully qualified staff and no possibility of intensive treatment otherwise. Therapists in Britain already frequently accept the patient's relatives in this role.

However in some parts of the country, volunteer schemes are already well established, many with the support of the Chest, Heart and Stroke Association (CHSA). Others have actually been set up by the local speech therapists themselves. Whatever the origins of such schemes it is vital that speech therapists make themselves available for advice and liaison and where possible give direct guidance to the volunteers. This is particularly important where dyspraxic patients are involved, as so much of the advice given out by the CHSA is aimed at those who are simply dysphasic.

Whatever a therapist's personal views on the use of volunteers, in many areas they are here to stay. If the speech therapy service in a locality is poorly staffed and under pressure, it is quite understandable that patients and anxious relatives will turn to whatever help is offered. The onus is thus on clinicians to help make such volunteer schemes successful for all those patients who wish to join them.

(g) Counselling of patient and relatives

Counselling is a vitally important aspect of treating the dyspraxic patient. The aims of the clinician in this respect will vary considerably, depending on the time which has elapsed since the cerebral trauma, the severity of the patient's communication problem and the likelihood of return to work and/or a near-normal life. As Wertz et al (1984) point out, counselling in the acute stage fulfils a different function from counselling of chronic apraxics, especially when the apraxia is severe.

Both patient and relatives usually want a return to the status quo prior to the CVA, however unrealistic this may be. For this reason they may be very reluctant at first even to consider alternative means of communication. They may not be ready to grasp the full implications of the patient's disorder in the early stages; and they tend to have only the haziest of ideas about what speech and language are, and how normal speech is produced. Furthermore, they may be unused to being in a hospital environment and have little idea of the time-scale involved in recovery from strokes or head injury and the likelihood of residual difficulties. They may even find the hemiplegia or other physical difficulties more devastating to cope with than the loss of speech, at least initially.

Counselling in the early stages, and with severe patients, means explaining to both patient and relatives what has gone wrong and why and outlining the general means of attempting to put things right. It means discussing the use of communication boards or of gestures or total communication. It means explaining such aspects as fatigue, emotional lability and depression. The patient's fluctuating abilities need to be put into perspective and understood by all before relatives can usefully participate in treatment, or even provide an appropriately encouraging communication environment at home. The difference between dysphasia and dyspraxia needs to be explained in layman's language and the patient's profile put over in simple terms so that both patient and relatives are aware of the difference between language stimulation and articulation therapy, and know which aspect predominates in their own case. Some of the specific techniques used for working on articulation may seem quite bizarre to patient and relatives initially. Therefore, in order to gain their cooperation, it is vital to explain simply the rationale for the use of such techniques as icing or phonetic derivation.

It is only fair that patient and relatives should be encouraged towards a realistic view of their future. This may be a gradual process and the skilled clinician does not try to hurry this period of adjustment. Team work, involving other members of the rehabilitation team, is just as vital in helping the patient and his relatives face the future as it is in other aspects of management, for the speech difficulties are unlikely to be his only problem. Coordinated counselling by doctors, physiotherapists, occupational therapists and particularly social workers, in addition to that provided by the speech therapist, may all be necessary over a period of time.

For the higher level patient where return to work is possible, counselling involves a different approach. The layman, be he patient, relative or employer, may find it hard to understand that recovery of any function (including speech) after brain damage, is not necessarily total. It is difficult for the public to grasp that someone can function well in one situation, such as home or clinic, yet find it hard to do as well in a crowded shop or busy office. Performance can be affected by fatigue, stress and other factors at this level of speech impairment just as at more severe levels; and 'off days' are not at all unusual. Even a cold may cause a temporary worsening of symptoms. Thus the mildly dyspraxic speaker may at times sound quite normal and at other times appear profoundly afflicted. The patient himself has to learn to accept and live within his limitations. His relatives and employer need to be aware that, to some extent, his normality is a veneer which is easily damaged if he is constantly under stress. Just as the dyspraxic talker learns to make adjustments, so too must his relatives and employer. Only in this way can optimum communication conditions be achieved.

Evaluation of the prognosis

In the previous section, some general issues affecting treatment of the dysphasic adult were considered. This section will examine more closely other important issues, with specific emphasis on the problems of the dyspraxic patient.

(a) General pointers

Just as there is still disagreement about the exact nature of apraxia of speech, there is also disagreement about the prognosis for patients who suffer from it. One reason for this is put forward by Rosenbek (1984):

'With few exceptions, data on the apraxic speaker's prognosis is buried in data on aphasia'.

Given that many dyspraxic patients also exhibit a degree of co-existing dysphasia, is it possible to separate the long-term effects of the two conditions? Rosenbek certainly thinks so:

'The presence of co-existing aphasia, its severity, and its improvement appeared to have no significant relationship with the presence, severity and improvement in apraxia of speech.'

Wertz et al (1984) discuss prognosis in some detail, comparing what we know about prognosis for aphasia with what we do or do not know about prognosis for apraxia. They advise some caution in using the prognostic variables applicable to aphasia for predicting change in apraxia, but agree that 'What we know about aphasia may be useful'. They find that no variables influencing recovery in apraxia of speech have stood up to rigorous examination but they rely on clinical experience and the literature on the subject to provide guidelines. On this basis, the patient with the best prognosis for recovery of speech is one with a small Broca's area lesion, who at a month or less post onset has minimal co-existing dysphasia, no oral apraxia, good health and plenty of stamina! They admit that such cases are rare and hence it is far more difficult to predict the future for the vast majority of dyspraxic patients.

(b) Specific guidelines

The above authors go on to look at other ways of making a prognosis. Under the heading of 'behavioural profiles' there is discussion of how PICA performance can be used predictively and of the value of Schuell's prognostic groups. For example, Schuell's minor syndrome B (aphasia with persisting dysfluency) has a much better prognosis than group 3 (aphasia with sensori-motor impairment). The former has an excellent prognosis for recovery of language but articulation may be variable, breaking down under stress, and automaticity and fluency are not regained (hence the term persisting dysfluency). The group 3 patient has a much more limited prognosis for both speech and language recovery but some functional use of language skills can be expected.

Wertz et al favour prognostic treatment as a means of finding out what the future holds and whether or not the patient is improving in response to treatment. Over a period of up to twenty treatment sessions (they use once or twice daily treatment as a rule), they systematically appraise four areas of interests which they describe in some detail. Four determinants are examined: improved performance on treated tasks, generalisation, retention, and willingness to practice. If all four determinants are positive, the prognosis with treatment is believed to be 'great'.

In practice, other general prognostic indicators including aetiology, size of lesion, localisation, health, severity and time of onset have all been found to have a significant effect on recovery from aphasia (Wertz et al, 1984). Education, pre-morbid intelligence, occupational status and type of aphasia play a more variable role; and the effects of such factors as sex, social mileu and motivation are even harder to define. Whether this is equally true for dyspraxia remains to be seen. However, we must keep all these factors in mind when we appraise the individual patient and his likely response to treatment. When we are satisfied that we have considered all the relevant prognostic indicators, we can formulate realistic goals for treatment.

Alternative methods of communication

When someone is speechless the immediate response of those around him may be to seek some other way in which they can communicate. Many a relative has thrust a pencil into a dysphasic patient's hand only to be very disappointed at the outcome. So it is with many of the more sophisticated alternatives available to the speech therapist. Many methods appear to hold out a great deal of promise, but few have so far proved wholly successful when applied in real life outside the clinical situation. Experience has shown that the patient who is predominantly dyspraxic rather than dysphasic may have more success in using methods with a verbal content such as writing or a communication board. The more severely dysphasic and dyspraxic patient is likely to need a simpler, less symbolic form of communication. The use of a manual system (gesture) is an attractive alternative but any patient with an ideomotor apraxia of the unparalysed arm would be likely to have difficulty using gesture. If the latter problem is severe, he may also have difficulty pointing and thus using a communication board.

(a) Visual systems

Recent interest has centred on two very different alternative methods of communication, the visual and the gestural. Bliss symbolics is the best known example of a visual symbol system and has undoubtedly been used successfully with cerebral palsied children; but its use with dysphasic and dyspraxic adults is less well documented. Stella Bailey presents a very interesting case study of work with one adult patient using Bliss symbols, in *Aphasia Therapy* (Code and Muller, 1983). Though her hopes for alleviating this patient's articulatory dyspraxia were not fulfilled, she feels that the results of her trial should 'encourage further investigation and more widespread use of Bliss with selected patients as an alternative treatment technique'.

A cautionary tale about the use and development of pictographic systems is told by Adrian Philpott in the *CST Bulletin* (October, 1985): in a study of 50 normal people interpreting the symbols used on the Convaid electronic speaking aid, over half the responses were wrong, nobody interpreted all the 112 pictograms correctly and 18 pictograms were interpreted wrongly by everyone!

Also in *Aphasia Therapy*, Rowley discusses the use of artificial languages in general and looks briefly at communication aids. He concludes that, in practice, artificial language systems may be of limited use outside the clinic unless technology can provide greater accessibility and comprehensibility for both patient and listener.

(b) New technology

In the same text, Enderby and Hamilton discuss the use of Splink (speech link) with 37 dysphasic patients, nine of whom were also dyspraxic or dysarthric. Splink is an electronic word board linked to a television screen by an infra-red transmitter (no wires) and containing 950 basic words, letters, numerals, common phrases, prefixes and suffixes. Enderby and Hamilton report that, of the 21 patients who mastered the use of Splink, all liked it but had required considerable help in learning to use it. Only nine patients found Splink useful in communication; twelve used it 'as an extension to therapy'; and it enabled eight of these to do homework (practising language tasks) which they would not otherwise have been able to do. The TV game aspect of Splink was seen as a motivator and encouraged more home practice. Since this study was reported other more sophisticated aids have become available but the same basic problem still applies – namely whether they will be utilised for effective communication.

The technology available for alternative communication systems is developing rapidly at the present time. Most of this progress relies on the availability of ever more powerful (and comparatively ever cheaper) micro-computers. The establishment of increasing numbers of regional Communication Aids Centres is essential if therapists are to have the opportunity to find out what systems are currently available. Some Health Authorities have already set up such centres where patients can be referred for assessment of their suitability for a variety of communication aids (*CST Bulletin*, March 1985).

The 'micro revolution' holds out a great deal of promise and it is easy to be dazzled or awed by such high technology. Undoubtedly it will be of enormous benefit to some people with impaired communication. The excellent BBC television series 'With a little help from the chip' and its accompanying booklet (Heddel, 1985) showed just how much can be done here and now. However, not all patients are willing or able to utilise this type of alternative method of communication and, as pointed out by Stella Bailey, 'there must be careful evaluation of the individual's abilities, needs and motivation.' It is essential that the family is also consulted as their encouragement is vital to success. Wertz et al (1984) remind clinicians of the difficulty of getting many patients to use even a simple communication board for real communication, in spite of the involvement of the family and ward personnel. This is something which most experienced clinicians will acknowledge.

(c) Gestural systems

It is tempting to see the use of gesture as a more acceptable alternative method of communication, and indeed many speechless patients spontaneously employ some gesture. However, those with an ideomotor apraxia of the unparalysed arm may find gesture extremely difficult if not impossible to learn. The current favourite gestural system for use with adult dyspraxics is Amerind, adapted for one-handed signing by Skelly (1974 and 1979). It has the advantage of being easily intelligible to the observer; and as it is not highly symbolic as sign languages are, even a patient with impaired ability to use language is able to make some progress with this system. The signs are very natural, eg. the person rubs his stomach with his hand to indicate hunger, and cups his hand to his ear to indicate the idea of hearing. Skelly found that, in addition to providing a means of communication, Amerind actually facilitated oral speech production.

Wertz et al discuss choosing an appropriate gestural system and methods of teaching it. They point out the value of including gesture in a 'total communication' programme where several modes of communication are worked on simultaneously.

Makaton is another gestural system which is popular with British therapists. Already Makaton groups for dysphasic and dyspraxic adults have been set up in certain parts of the country. Some have been running for a considerable time. Therapists have found the need to make changes to the Makaton system when using it with dysphasic patients. Initially a one-handed adaptation of the signing system was suggested (following the adaptation of Amerind for hemiplegic patients). However, in a discussion paper by Fay Thomson in 1981, it was suggested that there was no need to issue a standardized version of a one-handed system since, amongst other factors, there were few signs which could not be both formed and understood by using only half the sign. With regard to the vocabulary, it was felt that adults did not need to follow the developmental sequence but that the stages from concrete nouns to verbs to more abstract ideas were still relevant and useful. The basic vocabulary was felt to be adequate but adults would obviously need certain additions relevant to their environment.

One Makaton group brought to this author's attention, had two dyspraxic dysphasic patients and one with jargon dysphasia. It was felt by the therapist involved that Makaton helped all the patients in different ways. It improved comprehension for all, improved intelligibility in one patient, served as a vehicle for expression in two patients who could not speak or write, and generally increased sociability in the home. The conclusion reached was that signing using the Makaton vocabulary was a successful method of improving communication skills in these severely impaired stroke patients who had previously undergone a trial period of formal speech therapy and had made no significant improvement. This progress was achieved despite the fact that both dyspraxic patients also had an ideomotor apraxia of the unparalysed (left) hand which did affect the accuracy of their gestures and the ease with which they learned them.

An excellent study of the use of gesture and pantomime in the treatment of aphasia and apraxia is reported by Chris Code and Caroline Gaunt (1986).

The patient studied had severe aphasia and oral and limb apraxia 20 months post onset. Using a single case design (ABABA, where the A = testing and B = treatment), selected hand signs were taught from the Makaton vocabulary. In spite of the unpromising prognosis (based on the patient's severity, the time post onset and the amount of previous therapy and progress) objective testing showed that the patient had improved his ability to use a 'small range of useful hand signs'. However, it was admitted that this was a very limited result for a period of treatment spread over 8 months; and the clinicians were not aware of any carry-over or generalisation of the use of the learned gestures into spontaneous everyday communication situations.

From the above examples it can be seen that it is obviously well worth those clinicians who are trained in using either Amerind or Makaton introducing a gestural system to carefully selected dyspraxic patients. However, the patient and his family must be motivated to practise and use the system if it is to be of any real value for communication.

In August 1984, a specific interest group was set up in London to discuss the use of such non-verbal communication methods with dysphasic and dyspraxic adults (*CST Bulletin*, March 1985).

Summary

Whilst many of the issues discussed in this chapter are relevant to both dysphasic and dyspraxic patients – and particularly to those with combined disorders – Chapter 5 will concentrate on those techniques developed specifically to treat apraxia of speech. While the aim of this book is to provide practical information to help clinicians treat the majority of dyspraxic patients, ie. those who also have a coexisting degree of dysphasia, the emphasis will naturally be on the treatment of the dyspraxic element of the patient's disorder. This is not to undermine the importance of working on any concomitant dysphasia (often concurrently), as will be seen from the examples in Chapter 5 and the case studies in Chapter 6.

Chapter 5
METHODS OF TREATMENT

Proprioceptive neuromuscular facilitation /40
    (a) Stimulation /40
    (b) Manipulation /41
    (c) Case example/41

Articulatory diagrams /42
    (a) Development of the diagrams /42
    (b) Case example /42
    (c) Other visual techniques/43

Reauditorization /44
    (a) The rationale /44
    (b) The method /44
    (c) Case example/44

The use of prosody /45
    (a) Melodic intonation therapy /45
    (b) Case example /46
    (c) Contrastive stress drills /46
    (d) Four step programme /47
    (e) Gestural support/49

Rosenbek's 8 step continuum /50
    (a) Task selection /51
    (b) The eight steps/51

Other considerations /53
    (a) The need for continuous evaluation /53
    (b) Other aspects of treatment/54

CHAPTER 5
METHODS OF
TREATMENT

So far discussion has centred on the general issues relating to the treatment of the dyspraxic dysphasic patient. The aim of this section is to give a brief description of some of the special techniques currently in use in the treatment of articulatory dyspraxia. Amongst such techniques are proprioceptive neuro-muscular facilitation, the use of articulatory diagrams, reauditorization and the use of prosody. Rosenbek's 8-step continuum will also be described. The specific application of these techniques will be dealt with in more detail in Chapter 6.

Reports of new treatment programmes and task continua are continually being published and there is always a great deal of enthusiasm for new ideas. It is not suggested here that any one of these techniques or treatment programmes is to be used exclusively. In most cases an eclectic approach is to be preferred, with the therapist carefully monitoring the patient's responses to treatment and showing great flexibility in moving between techniques as appropriate. Some of the techniques make great demands on the patient's mental and physical stamina; and before the therapist embarks on a course of treatment, she must be satisfied that the amount of progress likely to be made justifies the amount of time and effort that both she and the patient will have to invest.

Proprioceptive neuromuscular facilitation

These techniques have been used extensively in the treatment of cerebral palsy and also with adult dysarthric patients. Some, though not all, of the PNF techniques have been tried with the severely dyspraxic or apraxic patient in an effort to bring buccofacial and articulatory movements under voluntary control. Methods of facilitation include stimulation and manipulation.

(a) Stimulation

Stimulation is the most popular when working with dyspraxics and usually takes the form of 'icing' and brushing (using a soft brush) to increase oral sensory awareness and stimulate movement. This can be used either indirectly, as when the alveolar ridge is stimulated to encourage elevation of the tongue, or directly, as when the muscle named orbicularis is stimulated by circular brushing or icing to facilitate pursing of the lips. The rationale for using icing techniques with apraxic patients is that the more severely impaired patients frequently have an oral sensory deficit where proprioception and tactile discrimination are affected. Since the neural pathways for the perception of temperature differ from those for touch and proprioception, one is hopefully utilizing a more intact pathway to provide sensory stimulation and feedback to compensate for poor position sense. The rationale for brushing is less clear. However it can be argued that anything which increases oral sensory awareness should help the apraxic patient to reorganise his oral and articulatory gestures. (It is not suggested that these techniques are of any value to the mildly or moderately dyspraxic speaker. Rather, they are often used as just part of the general stimulating and facilitating approach to bringing oral movements under voluntary control in patients who are severely dyspraxic or apraxic.)

The use of ice is potentially a messy business. However, problems can be minimised by holding an ice cube or crushed ice in a polythene bag or disposable surgical glove. Iced cotton wool buds can also be used, particularly when stimulating the velum. Hygiene is obviously an important factor to be considered here. There are two methods of icing: slow icing is helpful to reduce spasticity, and fast icing stimulates muscle tone. For the dyspraxic patient, icing is particularly helpful in facilitating perception of the position of the articulators, so either method may help – or even alternating methods.

(Caution is needed when applying ice, for it can burn. Five seconds icing is sufficient for each area, even when slow icing.)

Brushing can be carried out using a hand-held paint brush to stroke along the appropriate muscle prior to the required activity. Fast or rotary brushing can be carried out using a soft paint brush attached to a battery driven cocktail shaker or similar device (under 350 revolutions per minute is sufficient). Brushing is usually used to stimulate flaccid muscles and a time lag of 20 to 30 minutes can be expected between brushing and getting optimal results. The effect of icing is more immediate. It may therefore prove helpful to brush at the beginning of a treatment session, to do other work for 20 minutes, then to ice the same area before immediately carrying out the required movement exercises.

(b) Manipulation

Manipulation may also be used with apraxic patients. Direct manipulation of the articulators to the desired position is used by some, whilst others apply combinations of pressure, stretch and resistance, as described in the literature on PNF techniques. Pressure and stretch are used to facilitate movement, while resistance tends to be used only when the patient can make some unassisted movements of the appropriate muscles. Such resistance may be applied to the strong side while the weak side is assisted. Further details of these techniques and references to further reading about PNF can be found in Langley and Darvill (1979) on whose notes this section has been based. So far, the use of these techniques with apraxic patients has not been subjected to clinical trials. It would be very interesting to see if their popularity is deserved.

(c) Case example

This case is described more fully in Chapter 6. Mrs M was found to have very severe dyspraxia and icing was used as a means of facilitation. An ice cube, wrapped in a paper tissue, was applied to the upper and lower lips with a quick, light, stroking movement in an attempt to make her more aware of the position of these articulators. Articulation work in the session was concentrating on the production of /m/ in conjunction with /ɑ/ aiming for maximum contrast of lip closed and open positions, whilst utilizing the vibration accompanying production of /m/ for additional reinforcement of the lips closed position. /m/ was also the consonant selected because it could be derived from humming.

However, attempts to sequence /m/ with a vowel (either CV of VC) led to great frustration and production of associated or even unrelated articulatory movements, eg. tongue protrusion. Use of a mirror did not help this patient but manipulation of the articulators did. Icing of the lips was thus used as an intermediate step between manipulation and voluntary lip closure and opening. The use of icing and the 'feel' of the position of the ice cold lips, was not the only facilitation involved. In fact it was embedded in a great many other stimulating and facilitating procedures which will be described in Chapter 6.

Articulatory diagrams

(a) Development of the diagrams

Luria (1970) first popularized the use of articulatory diagrams (sometimes known as articulograms) in his treatment of afferent and efferent motor aphasia. Since both these syndromes can be viewed as aphasia with a degree of articulatory dyspraxia, synonymous with Schuell's group 3 and minor syndrome B patients respectively, the technique has frequently been applied when patients have a severe degree of articulatory dyspraxia. The diagrams are often used to reinforce articulatory movements derived from direct manipulation, phonetic derivation, and 'listen and watch me' approaches. They are a tangible and visual 'sound form' which the patient can refer back to, unlike other more fleeting stimuli. Where use of a mirror helps the patient, he can even help himself with his homework using articulatory diagrams. They are useful at the most basic level of eliciting and reinforcing single phonemas in VC or CV combinations and also in building to more complex syllables and sound clusters. Where relatives are helping directly in the patient's treatment, they can provide very explicit guidelines to carry over practice from clinic to home.

Examples of the type of diagram which has been found clinically useful can be found in the Appendices. These are based on diagrams which were produced to the author's specifications by graphic artist J Cameron in 1976. He designed two master copies which could be photo-copied and used in many different ways depending on the patient's needs. The clear black-and-white diagrams were felt to be more useful than photographs as the desired position of the articulators could easily be emphasised and the voicing feature indicated. The latter was done by the use of a zig-zag line drawn below the lips. Nasality was indicated in a similar way, with the zig-zag printed above the lips.

(b) Case example

Mrs M above also benefitted from the use of articulatory diagrams. Very early on in treatment, individual diagrams were used to reinforce single consonants and vowels being worked on. As soon as any sequencing of VC or CV combinations was attempted, the diagrams were utilized to reinforce what was wanted. The example previously cited, of eliciting and sequencing /ɑ/ and /m/ using PNF techniques, was followed up with the production of sounds to stimulation by the therapist (listen and watch me) with the added visual reinforcement of the diagrams. Later, Mrs M achieved production to the stimulus of the diagrams alone; and eventually the stimulus of the written word 'arm' (or a picture of an arm) sufficed to elicit the desired utterance. This was followed up by 'closure' exercises and forced alternatives to reinforce the sounds as real words in a linguistic context as follows:

- **Therapist:** Let me take your . . . (points to patient's arm).
  Patient: Arm.
- **Therapist:** A leg and an . . . (tapping or pointing to patient's body part as appropriate).
  Patient: Arm.
- **Therapist:** Raise your . . . (helping patient to do the action).
  Patient: Arm.
- **Therapist:** Wave your . . . (helping patient do the action).
  Patient: Arm.
- **Therapist:** I've hurt my . . . (miming).
  Patient: Arm.

In addition the word 'arm' was included in comprehension and auditory discrimination exercises and Mrs M practised writing the word and doing written sentence completion exercises for homework. The articulatory diagrams had the added benefit of being very useful reinforcers for homework use and Mr M, who sat in on most treatment sessions, found they helped him to help his wife in the same way.

(c) Other visual techniques

It seems appropriate at this point to mention the use of two other visual techniques – mirror-work and video tapes. Mirror-work tends to be unpopular for a variety of reasons. Some clinicians do not like it as they feel it discourages the patient, especially in the early stages, if he is confronted by his altered appearance (Wertz, 1984). Others find that it is not nearly as effective as using the therapist as a model. Often severely dyspraxic patients will inspect their teeth and tidy their hair when confronted with a mirror, rather than watch themselves producing sounds. Patient T described in Chapter 6 is an example of this. It seems that people quite naturally do not like to see themselves 'pulling funny faces'. According to Rosenbek, Darley actually cites as one of his 13 characteristics of apraxia of speech that, 'articulatory performance is unaffected by . . . availability of visual monitoring by mirror' (Rosenbek, 1984). It therefore seems unlikely that a mirror would be of any great value beyond the stage of production of simple CVC combinations, but there will always be some patients who do benefit from some mirror-work at some point alongside other facilitating techniques.

The use of video in this context is fairly new and little has been written about it. Wertz et al dislike the use of a video monitor as much as they dislike mirror-work. However, imaginative use of videotapes of treatment made by the therapist for use by the patient at home is a different proposition. A case was reported to the author where a young, highly motivated single male with severe dyspraxia was able to do considerable home practice using videotapes made of his sessions with his speech therapist. (The video machine he used at home was loaned by his employers.) Since a significant percentage of homes now possess video playback machines, their use in this way becomes a possibility for more than just an enthusiastic minority. This patient's therapist reported very much better progress than she might otherwise have expected, suggesting that it is well worth researching the effect on treatment of video used in this way.

Reauditorization

(a) The Rationale

If apraxia of speech is seen as a purely motor speech problem, the rationale for using any auditory stimulation technique seems rather controversial. However, Wertz et al point out that 'motor planning requires sensory-motor integrations', so that even in a patient with a pure articulatory dyspraxia there may be some theoretial basis for eg. auditory discrimination training. In practice, it is rarely deemed appropriate unless the patient is also dysphasic. The value of auditory training and stimulation when the patient is both dysphasic and dyspraxic, is less in doubt. In fact Schuell was a great advocate of 'intensive controlled auditory stimulation', otherwise known as reauditorization, for patients with little or no functional speech, and described it as the method of choice for patients with severe sensorimotor impairment ie. dysphasic patients who are also severely dyspraxic (Schuell, 1964).

Wertz et al report that various studies have been carried out recently on many other aspects of auditory stimulation eg. use of white noise and DAF (delayed auditory feedback) with dyspraxic speakers. The use of imposed rhythms such as by metronome or using Melodic Intonation Therapy (MIT) has also been examined, but it appears that none of these studies have specifically covered those aspects of auditory stimulation advocated by Schuell.

(b) The method

Reauditorization involves the use of the visual as well as the auditory modality – but the emphasis is on getting the patient to *listen*, initially to the clinician's stimulus and then to his own response as well. The primary objective is to enable the patient 'to hear and think the word', and to this end the clinician repeats the word about 20 times. The interval between repetitions needs to be long enough to allow the patient to 'rehearse' the word and eventually say it. If he struggles to produce the word he is directed to listen again. The aim is to teach 20 items (pictured words) each week (assuming a daily therapy session). Although the method was initially designed for use by the clinician with the patient, a Language Master can be used once the patient becomes able to repeat with ease.

(c) Case example

Once again Mrs M serves as a useful case example. Since this patient was only receiving treatment once weekly only a limited vocabulary was utilized. The reauditorization technique was introduced once Mrs M became able to produce some words voluntarily and on imitation. Until this point, repetition was quite beyond her and virtually every utterance required the use of other facilitating techniques. Words which were within her capability when more directly facilitated were chosen. Only two were attempted in any session. As perseveration was often a problem, the words chosen were very different, eg. 'arm' and 'tea', to minimize articulatory and semantic confusion. At one point a Language Master was introduced in the hope that she could make use of this in home practice; but unfortunately Mrs M and high technology did not interact well. The machine threw her into a panic because everything happened much too fast! After a trial period, it was decided that her husband was a much more acceptable substitute as a stimulus.

The use of prosody

A completely different facilitatory technique, and one which is of more value with the less impaired patient, is the use of prosody as an aid to fluency. The most extreme form of this technique is Melodic Intonation Therapy (Sparks and Holland, 1979) which has been used with severely dysphasic patients, for whom the technique was developed, but which is of debatable value to patients who are purely dyspraxic.

(a) Melodic Intonation Therapy

Sparks and Holland describe a structured programme appropriate for both individual and group treatment. The method utilizes the patient's remaining musical ability (assuming he has any) and is only suitable for those who have retained the ability to sing familiar material. The best candidates for this type of therapy according to Sparks are Broca's aphasics (Wernicke's aphasics are definitely not suitable). The rationale is that the potential of the preserved right hermisphere is tapped to facilitate the return of spoken language. As with many current treatment approaches, a rigorous programme is suggested for using MIT. Suitable candidates are guided through four different levels of therapy, starting at level I where the clinician establishes a set of singing and tapping rhythms based on short meaningful phrases and sentences. (The intonation patterns and melodies of these phrases are worked out in advance by the clinician.) At the first level the patient and therapist hum the melody in unison and tap the rhythm together. At level II the patient initially just listens to the stimulus, then he attempts to join in so that patient and therapist chant in unison. The therapist then fades her voice out but continues tapping the rhythmn as the patient continues intoning. Next the clinician intones the phrase and the patient repeats it, accompanied by tapping. Finally the clinician asks him to repeat what he just said, which he does, tapping out the rhythm. Each step of the procedure is scored and it is discontinued at any step after failure (ie. less than 90% success).

Level III follows a similar pattern to level II but progresses more quickly through intoning and tapping in unison, to repetition and tapping by the patient, to a question intoned by the clinician with the patient producing an appropriate response. At level IV the clinician intones the stimulus which the patient repeats after a delay (tapping continues). Both then intone in unison and the clinician fades out her voice. The clinician presents the intoned sentence again and the patient repeats it, continuing to tap the rhythm. Then the clinician presents the sentence using normal prosody and the patient repeats it in normal speech. Finally the clinician asks a question which the patient answers with the practice phrase or sentence or similar, in normal speech.

The sorts of phrases suggested, with their melodic line, are as follows:

7 o'clock	se	ven	o'	clock	
take a shower	take	a	sho	wer	
it is lunch time	it	is	lunch	time	
I want a drink	I	want	a	drink	
a nice cup of tea	a	nice	cup	of	tea

According to Wertz et al this method is unproven with dyspraxic patients and they even go so far as to say 'Imposing melodic intonation or DAF seems to erode articulatory performance'. However, when a patient is both dysphasic and dyspraxic, especially if the dysphasia is the primary problem, then there is some justification for using the technique. It is certainly a technique which has interested therapists in the past; and many claim to have tried it in a modified form with their severely dysphasic and dyspraxic patients, though as yet no case studies have been reported. Some therapists feel that it gives the patient confidence and that the strong rhythmic element is useful in helping the patient keep to a slow syllabic pace. Used in this way it can be an exaggerated prosodic facilitator and can lead on to more natural prosodic drills. The MIT programme includes the use of tapping rhythms along with intoning and this type of gestural support for prosody is described later for use with less severely dyspraxic patients.

(b) Case example

Mr G had very severe dyspraxia and dysphasia. Initially he had no speech at all and could not even vocalize. Treatment was approached on several fronts, including the use of MIT-like exercises with simultaneous tapping. The rhythmic element was observed to help speech production. Direct articulation work was also pursued doggedly with new CV and VC combinations being steadily introduced, building a small spoken vocabulary of useful words. Gesture and writing were also encouraged.

(c) Contrastive stress drills

Also making use of prosodic features is the contrastive stress drill described by Wertz et al. This procedure requires that the patient has speech and is therefore most appropriate for the mildly or moderately dyspraxic patient where poor articulation is the primary problem. The rationale for using contrastive stress drills is that articulation is facilitated by primary stress, so forced alternative and question-and-answer techniques can be used to structure the patient's speech output, forcing the desired sound or sound combinations into a stressed position in his responses. For example, if the target is word initial /p/ the word 'pie' can be drilled in the following way. The therapist explains to the patient what the target sound is and the word to be drilled, and that this will be done using a question-and-answer dialogue. They then proceed as follows:

- **Therapist:** Did you eat steak?
  Patient: No, *pie*.
- **Therapist:** Do you want curry?
  Patient: I want *pie*.
- **Therapist:** Pie or cheese?
  Patient: *Pie*.
- **Therapist:** Did you want pork curry?
  Patient: No, a *pork pie*.

Examples of drills for all word initial consonants are given in Appendix IV. It is hoped these may provide a useful starting point for clinicians to build specific exercises for individual patients.

The general principles for using such drills are as follows. Firstly, the drill is built around just one or a very few target sounds embedded in a sentence made up of easily articulated sounds. Secondly, the target must be a sound which the patient can sometimes produce normally, or very nearly so. This type of drill does not facilitate correct production of an aberrant sound but it does encourage wider use of sounds which the patient can produce in more limited contexts. Thirdly, word and utterance length have to be rigorously controlled and kept well within the patient's capability. Fourthly, the place of the target in the word, and the word in the utterance, need to be carefully thought out since some locations are easier for dyspraxics than others. Finally, the matrix of the utterance (ie. the sounds in which the target is embedded) must be sounds which the patient can already produce easily. For example, if the target is /t/ and only vowels are available, the therapist is limited to drilling such words as tea, toe, eat, art, etc. If the patient can also easily produce the sounds /p/ and /m/ this list can be extended to include pat, tap, mat, tame, pot, etc. The difficulty of constructing drills of suitable words quite clearly limits the use of such drills to more able patients, and makes them inappropriate for those with a gross problem.

(d) Four-step programme

Wertz et al also describe a four-step programme by which a sound combination can progress from imitation, through question-and-answer to use in spontaneous speech. The imitation step involves the use of a 'slow motion speech' model by the clinician and its imitation by the patient. The second step begins with an explanation to the patient of what is required and why. The clinician gives the patient his practice utterance (in appropriate answer format) then asks appropriate questions to elicit that answer. The third step makes the drill more difficult, either by changing the stimuli or by changing the criteria for success. The fourth step expands and modifies the drill further, using a carefully constructed question-and-answer game. For example, if the therapist is aiming to improve the consonant blend /pl/ in a word initial position, a discourse going through the following stages might be appropriate:

Step 1. Imitation

■ **Therapist:** I want you to say what I say . . . (very slowly and deliberately whilst facing the patient) . . . /pələ, pələ, pələ/
Patient: /pələ, pələ, pələ/

■ **Therapist:** Good! Now this time we will put the sound /pl/ into the word 'play'. Listen and copy me . . . (again slowly and deliberately) . . . /pəleɪ, pəleɪ/
Patient: /pəleɪ, pəleɪ/

■ **Therapist:** Fine. Now this time I want you to run the sounds together and say the word a little quicker, like this . . . (slowly but without the intrusive schwa) . . . /pleɪ, pleɪ/
Patient: /pəleɪ, pleɪ/

■ **Therapist:** Not bad. Let's have it again . . . /pleɪ/
Patient: /pleɪ/

■ **Therapist:** Good. You are doing well.

Step 2. Question and answer format.

■ **Therapist:** OK, now I want you to use the word 'play' as the answer to some questions. This time, you are not saying it after me but you are using the word as an answer. So if I say 'What do you see at the theatre?'

you can answer 'A play'. Do you follow the idea?
Patient nods.

- **Therapist:** Right, let's try. Would you rather see a film or a play?
  Patient: A play.

- **Therapist:** What's on at the theatre?
  Patient: A play.

- **Therapist:** Is the Mousetrap a famous film?
  Patient: A famous play.

Step 3. Making the drill more difficult.

Here the patient is expected to use the word being drilled in response to different stimuli. As the drill progresses, he is encouraged to produce a clearer and better response.

- **Therapist:** Fine. Now this time we'll do it in a different way. I still want you to use the word 'play', but sometimes it will be 'plays' or 'playing' or 'played'. First I want you to read some words (presents cards with those words written, one at a time, for the patient to read out loud).
  Patient reads the cards out loud.

- **Therapist:** Good. Now this time I want you to concentrate hard on the /pl/ sound and do it as well as you can . . .

Step 4. Further expansion of the drill using question-and-answer format.

- **Therapist:** Well done. Now this time we are going to use the /pl/ words again as answers to questions. First of all I'll show you some pictures and ask you about them; but remember the answer is one of those /pl/ words . .
    (shows appropriate pictures) . . . What are the children doing?
  Patient: Playing.

- **Therapist:** What is the man doing?
  Patient: Playing golf.

- **Therapist:** Is he playing the stroke or has he just played it?
  Patient: Just played it.

- **Therapist:** Right. That was good. Let's move on to some more questions and answers, without the pictures this time. Remember we are still using the word 'play' as part of the answer and concentrating on the /pl/ sound, getting it clear and smooth. This time I want you to put the word 'play' into a sentence too. Do you play poker?
  Patient: No, I don't play poker.

- **Therapist:** What do you like to play?
  Patient: I like to play whist.

- **Therapist:** Have you seen any good plays on TV?
  Patient: I don't watch plays on TV.

- **Therapist:** Do you like to play panel games?
  Patient: Yes, I like to play panel games.

The scope for role play at this juncture is considerable, if the therapist and patient find it a useful practical medium. As can be seen from this lengthy example, the later stages of the drill require the patient to be a comparatively competent speaker and are well beyond the capability of more severely dyspraxic patients, particularly those who are also dysphasic.

Further details and examples of this approach can be found in Wertz et al. As mentioned before, this method is only suitable for generalizing the production of sounds and sound combinations which the patient can already produce fairly easily.

(e) Gestural support

As an adjunct to teaching contrastive stress drills, Wertz et al include a section on the use of illustrative gesture to enhance such drills. The illustrative gestures they advocate are 'baton' movements and rhythmic pacing movements. They describe an eight-step programme for teaching the use of such a 'tapping and talking' approach, but recognize that such a new and experimental procedure needs to be carefully explained to the patient. It is claimed that those patients who can tap out simple rhythms and link those rhythms to speaking, are providing themselves with extra cues to speech (along the lines of Luria's intersystemic reorganisation). The rhythmic gestures are specifically linked with contrastive stress drills. However, they are not intended to be used indefinitely (though some patients do) but rather as a temporary facilitator of rhythmic awareness in speech. The final step in the programme is to fade out the use of gesture. They also describe the use of a pacing board, a piece of apparatus the patient can walk his fingers along, as an aid to gestural pacing.

For higher level patients, Wertz suggests expanding the contrastive stress drill to make it more challenging. Longer words and sentences can be used, sentences may be loaded with more targets and less common words, and a faster speaking rate can be encouraged. The clinician can give fewer cues and may even interrupt to add realism to the dialogue. Stimuli can be more natural with emphasis on stress, rhythm and sentence length rather than on specific sounds and syllables. Six methods of varying the contrastive stress drills are described, as are methods of strengthening the patient's responses. Reading aloud is considered a useful adjunct to therapy at this level.

A similar procedure is described by Fawcus, Robinson, Williams, J and Williams, R (1983) in *Working with Dysphasics*, and extensive examples of suitable exercises can be found in their text. However, the emphasis is on word retrieval rather than the generalization of specific sounds. They also suggest the use of beating out the desired pattern, initially syllable-timing, then beating out the stressed syllables. This is directly comparable to the use of tapping as an illustrative gesture (just described) and bears some similarity to the approach used in Melodic Intonation Therapy. Patients can be drilled on two, three and four-syllable words so that they beat out the stress pattern as they speak the word. They suggest similar use of reading aloud, and eliciting the desired word by appropriate questions.

Example

The patient is given a word of 2, 3, or 4 syllables to practise, depending on his capability, and the syllables are marked. The word is presented orally and visually and the patient is asked to say the target word, stressing all the syllables.

2 syllables

<u>Lon</u>	<u>don</u>	<u>tea</u>	<u>pot</u>
<u>Do</u>	<u>ver</u>	<u>car</u>	<u>pet</u>

3 syllables:

<u>Mar</u> <u>ga</u> <u>ret</u>   <u>com</u> <u>pu</u> ter

<u>vi</u> <u>de</u> <u>o</u>   <u>ra</u> <u>di</u> <u>o</u>

4 syllables:

<u>te</u> <u>le</u> <u>vi</u> <u>sion</u>   <u>po</u> <u>li</u> <u>ti</u> <u>cian</u>

He is then asked to beat out the syllables of the target word, emphasizing the normal stress pattern:

<u>tea</u> pot

com <u>pu</u> tor

<u>te</u> le vi sion

The normal prosodic pattern may also be targetted:

téa pòt

com pú tòr

tél è vi sion.

The practice word is then introduced into a stressed position in a short sentence which the patient reads aloud:

<u>London</u>   is our capital city.

<u>Video</u>   games are fun.

<u>Television</u>   wastes time.

The next stage is to elicit the target word using question-and-answer techniques and finally to attempt to elicit the word in spontaneous speech (eg. picture description or discussion of a set topic).

Such prosodic aids can also be used to build up syllable sequences and they give many useful examples such as:

foot, football, footballer

These can be read aloud, spoken with a beat and elicited in response to appropriate questions. The authors also go on to give examples of other aspects of articulation drills not so dependant on prosody, eg. drilling two syllable words with a constant first syllable, and three syllable words with two first syllables constant:

convict, convent

underpin, undermine

Rosenbek's eight-step continuum

A systematic approach to the treatment of less severely impaired patients was put forward by Rosenbek, Lemme, Ahern, Harris and Wertz (1973) and was later modified by Deal and Florence (1978). In the original paper, the emphasis was on a carefully structured and graded set of drills to be used both intensively and extensively, aiming at meaningful communication as early as possible, and at efficient self-correction. This programme concentrates on the disordered articulation, unlike Schuell's much broader language-based approach, and takes into account factors known about the order of difficulty of articulatory production in apraxia of speech.

(a) Task selection

Tasks are arranged hierarchically from easiest through to hardest (eg. vowels, nasals and plosives before fricatives and affricatives; singletons before consonant clusters; word final before word initial sounds). It is important that the patient achieves success each session and does not have to struggle, hence the need for very careful stimulus selection. As sound sequencing becomes possible, the aim is to increase the distance gradually between points of articulation. (This is in direct contrast to the approach often needed in the early stages with very severe dyspraxia, where individual sounds worked on need to be maximally different to avoid perseveration.)

Both auditory and visual stimulation are emphasised, ie. integral stimulation epitomised as 'listen and watch me'. As the patient progresses, first auditory then visual cues are faded out. Only if integral stimulation fails do Rosenbek et al advocate using phonetic placement (manipulating the articulators), phonetic derivation (eg. eliciting a /m/ from humming) or 'key word' methods (using a key word which the patient can say to get him to produce the desired sound in other words and contexts).

(b) The eight steps

The original task continuum progresses through eight steps, outlined below, though the modified continuum omits some stages when patients are successful.

Step 1
'Listen and watch me' (integral stimulation) with the therapist providing the stimulus.

Step 2
After integral stimulation and a slight delay, the patient imitates the target. The therapist gives a visual (mouthed) cue, fading the auditory cue.

Step 3
The cues are dropped so that the task is one of simple imitation.

Step 4
There is integral stimulation by the therapist, then successive productions by the patient with no further stimulus or cues. (Later trials in fact showed this step to be more difficult than later steps, and therefore possibly misplaced.)

Step 5
Here the stimulus is written and production is simultaneous ie. reading aloud.

Step 6
The stimulus is written but production is delayed, putting a heavier load on memory.

Step 7

The imitative model is abandoned and the target elicited by a question.

Step 8

The target is produced in role play.

Therapists are advised to present stimuli slowly with pauses between words or groups of words, increased stress and exaggerated articulatory gestures. When a patient has particular difficulty, prolongation of consonants and vowels and the use of an intrusive schwa with consonant clusters is suggested. The effect of this is to produce a slow motion speech model. An example of how this programme might be put into action can be seen below.

(c) Example

Here the therapist is drilling the word 'tea' following the steps just outlined:

Step 1

■ **Therapist:** Listen and watch me.

'Tea, tea, tea.'

Step 2

■ **Therapist:** Now this time, I want you to listen then copy what I say. Listen and watch me . . . 'tea, tea, tea'.
Patient: (much groping) /pi, fpi/ (therapist mouths cues) /ti/.

■ **Therapist:** Not bad, but let's try it again. (This step is completed successfully on the second attempt.)

Step 3

■ **Therapist:** Now I want you to say 'tea' after me. I shall say it three times, but you just say it once.

'Tea,   tea,   tea.'
Patient: /ti/

Step 4

■ **Therapist:** That was good. This time I want you to listen and watch me then say 'tea' three times without any more help. Listen and watch me . . . 'tea'.
Patient: /ti, ti, ti/

Step 5

■ **Therapist:** You are doing well. Here is the word we have been working on, written down. Can you read this (presents word card)?
Patient: (reads) 'Tea'.

Step 6

■ **Therapist:** That was fine. Now this time I will show you the word, then

52

take it away. Then you say it (shows word card then removes it).
Patient: 'Uh! tea.'

Step 7

■ **Therapist:** Good. Now I want you to use the word 'tea' as the answer when I ask you a question. 'Do you like coffee or tea?'
Patient: 'Tea'.

■ **Therapist:** (making it more difficult) 'What would you like to drink?'
Patient: Tea.

Step 8

■ **Therapist:** This is going very well. OK, this time I want you to imagine you are in a cafe and you want a cup of tea. I'll be the counter assistant . . .

Up to this point the example given could be of a severely dyspraxic patient being drilled on one of a very limited number of words. However, the introduction of role play is obviously aimed at much higher level patients. The more speech and language a patient has, the more flexible and interesting the drill and the easier it can be to devise appropriate role play. With a mildly dyspraxic patient the therapist would be expecting a much higher standard of performance of the target.

Rosenbek et al do not see this approach as guaranteed to produce success and are quite realistic about the time and effort involved. However, they feel that the use of this approach will 'help restore some communicative ability to some severely apraxic patients'. They go on to say that therapy for apraxia of speech is 'a painfully long gruelling process' and concede that where the patient has to pay for his treatment, it may be prohibitively expensive.

Wertz et al echo these sentiments on the cost-effectiveness of therapy, both in financial terms and in terms of what the patient gains from the effort he is required to put into therapy. However, though they emphasize the need for the use of treatment hierarchies or task continua, they also stress the need for great flexibility. Treatment is dynamic and must respond to the patient's successes.

Other considerations

(a) The need for continuous evaluation

There is no doubt that clinicians are under increasing pressure to show that their methods work, particularly in countries where the patient or his insurance company must pay directly for his treatment. However it should always be a basic principle of treatment that proven methods of treatment should be first choice, and that unproven techniques must be carefully and continuously monitored until their value is established (or otherwise). Only after such careful evaluation can we confidently disregard techniques which offer little return, concentrating our efforts on those which will effect improvement so long as other prognostic indicators are favourable. Many of the techniques described here have yet to be validated in clinical trials and their popularity ratified. Given this situation it would seem advisable for every clinician to carry out her own treatment trials, using single case designs if necessary, until such time as larger-scale longer-term studies demonstrate the efficacy or otherwise of favoured treatment methods.

Wertz et al suggest the use of three types of single case design: the withdrawal or ABA design, the multiple baseline design and the alternating treatments design. Both general and specific guidelines are given for their use with dyspraxic patients. However the emphasis is on articulation drills, and though this subject is dealt with in some detail, the method is not generalized to other aspects of therapy with patients who are both dysphasic and dyspraxic. A more general discussion of single case designs in the treatment of dysphasia is provided by Max Coltheart in *Aphasia Therapy* (Code and Muller, 1983). Here, it is suggested that such single case studies are actually of more value in demonstrating the efficacy of treatment than are larger-scale group studies, where subtle effects may become lost in the statistical analysis of broader changes.

(b) Other aspects of treatment

A general discussion of the principles of treatment can be found in *Apraxia of Speech in Adults: the Disorder and its Management*, by Wertz et al (1984). Apraxia treatment is compared with that for dysphasia and dysarthria and there is discussion of sensory modalities (auditory, tactile/kinaesthetic and visual) and their use in the treatment of apraxia. The efficiency of treatment is also considered and a guide to the selection and ordering of stimuli presented, once again very much geared to work on articulation drills. Such aspects as frequency of occurrence of sounds, position in a word, ease of stimulation (stimulability), occurrence in connected speech and exploitation of distinctive features are all covered. The importance of pairing stimuli, to establish phonemic contrasts early in therapy, is discussed and the effects of generalization considered.

Both Wertz and Rosenbek emphasize the importance of using hierarchical task continua. Rosenbek summarizes numerous recent studies examining such things as modality of stimulation, response conditions, and imitation delay and rehearsal. He also describes studies into the use of special methods either directly or indirectly affecting speech. Examples of the former range from the use of electromyography assisted biofeedback (a research technique which few therapists are likely to have encountered) to simply altéring the communication environment. Examples of the latter include the use of a metronome, delayed auditory feedback, vibrotactile stimulation and gestures, fuller details of which can be found in the above-mentioned publications.

CHAPTER 6
TREATMENT:
APPLICATION OF
TECHNIQUES

Categories of apraxic patients /56

    (a) Gross disorder /56

    (b) Very severe disorder /57

    (c) Severe disorder /57

    (d) Moderate disorder /57

    (e) Mild to moderate disorder /58

    (f) Mild disorder /58

    (g) Minimal disorder./58

Treatment /58

    (a) Treatment of gross disorder /59

    (b) Treatment of very severe disorder /62

    (c) Treatment of severe disorder /65

    (d) Treatment of moderate disorder /66

    (e) Treatment of mild to moderate disorder /68

    (f) Treatment of mild disorder /70

    (g) Treatment of minimal disorder/71

Chapter 6
TREATMENT: APPLICATION OF TECHNIQUES

In the previous chapter a wide range of popular methods used with dyspraxic patients were reviewed in a general way. The purpose of this chapter is to describe the application of those principles and methods of treatment to the types of patients most frequently encountered in our clinics. It is therefore relevant at this point to describe in some detail the variety of dyspraxic patients we see and to attempt to categorize them in a way which makes selection of appropriate treatment techniques easier.

Categories of apraxic patients

Most dyspraxic adults appearing in our clinics will also have a coexisting degree of dysphasia of varying severity at some stage in their recovery if not permanently. Some will be mildly dysphasic and severely dyspraxic, some exactly the reverse, and many will have similar degrees of severity of both disorders. For ease of handling information, patients have been divided here into eight categories based primarily on the severity of the dyspraxia but recognizing the frequent co-occurrence of varying degrees of dysphasia. Thus the categories also reflect the overall degree of communication problem presented by patients who are both dyspraxic and dysphasic. This does not mean that an isolated dyspraxia, sometimes of considerable severity, does not exist; rather that such pure apraxia is not encountered very frequently.

The categories used are derived from observation of the author's and other patients over a period of years. They are descriptive and may be applied to patients at different stages in their recovery as well as describing how they initially present early after CVA. For this reason the comments on prognosis must obviously be interpreted in the light of the diagnostic category the patient is in relative to the time since onset, eg. a patient with a very severe disorder in the early stages should do better than one in the same category at a year post onset.

(a) Gross disorder

This is the most severely affected category and the one with the poorest prognosis for recovery of speech and language. The patient is generally speechless and may be quite unable to communicate in any way initially. He may have a severe bucco-facial apraxia and severe or even global aphasia. Since he has no speech, the diagnosis of apraxia of speech has to be made with some caution (Wertz, 1984). He is probably hemiplegic and he may also have a degree of ideomotor apraxia affecting his unparalysed hand, hence he may be unable to use gesture to communicate even if his symbolic skills are adequate. Many patients may appear this severely affected in the first hours or days after cerebral trauma but spontaneous recovery often results in dramatic improvement. If however, after the first month the patient is still equally impaired, the outlook is obviously poor. A period of diagnostic therapy may be necessary to discover if the patient has any potential for recovery of speech or language, or for learning an alternative method of communication.

(b) Very severe disorder

Though patients in this group make virtually no spontaneous speech attempts, they may be able to cooperate with some bucco-facial and oral tasks. However many have a severe oral apraxia making it difficult to cooperate with direct work on articulation in the early stages. They are usually at least moderately dysphasic but this can be variable. Right hemiplegia is usual and left-limb apraxia may also be present. Treatment sessions tend to concentrate on improving the dysphasia since attempts to work on speech can result in extreme frustration for both patient and clinician. However in many cases it is well worth attempting some articulation work, preferably in short bursts at regular intervals. A great deal of sensory stimulation and feedback is required as the patient often has poor proprioceptive abilities and sometimes inadequate auditory monitoring (Jenkins et al, 1975). Alternative methods of communication might be considered as a temporary aid or for use to support speech on a permanent basis (Wertz et al, 1984). A great deal of flexibility is needed in dealing with patients so severely impaired and to some extent treatment continues to be diagnostic for some time as the clinician explores all useful channels of communication and means of facilitating production of speech. (Wertz et al describe this approach as 'total communication'). The speech prognosis may be very limited for these patients but it can be argued that a little speech is better than none at all. Since the effort involved in regaining limited speech is enormous, the patient and relatives need to be given a realistic prognosis as soon as possible and allowed to participate in decisions about how long to continue with treatment. The therapist's responsibility for providing sensitive counselling and support is a key issue here.

(c) Severe disorder

Patients in this category usually attempt to speak, though what they produce is severely limited, laboured and difficult to understand. Again there is often at least a moderate degree of coexistent dysphasia though this is not always the case. Because the patient has some speech it is easier to differentiate the dyspraxic and dysphasic elements of his disorder. He may also have a right hemiplegia and a degree of left ideomotor apraxia. The prognosis for recovery of speech in this group (all other variables being favourable) is generally better than for the previous two categories, as the patient is better able to cooperate with the work needed on articulation. The generally higher level of language skills also allows greater variety and flexibility in treatment. He is less likely to need, or to want to use, alternative methods of communication though he may benefit from the temporary use of techniques appropriate to the more severely impaired. Once again, the clinician must be extremely flexible and judge carefully if this is necessary.

(d) Moderate disorder

Since these patients present speaking, the task of diagnosing the presence of articulatory dyspraxia is made considerably easier. Their utterances are often slow and laboured, and they may display a foreign sounding accent. Prosody can be greatly disrupted, with intelligibility breaking down at times. The degree of accompanying dysphasia may be very variable and these patients may be able to write better than they can talk. They do communicate using speech, however haltingly, and are unlikely to wish to use any alternative methods of communication. The prognosis for improved speech is variable as progress is still hard won, and the patient's motivation to work on his speech can be a deciding factor.

(e) Mild to moderate disorder

For these patients, speech is the primary mode of communication even if it is often slow and effortful. The accompanying dysphasia may be very mild so that the listener is primarily aware of the disrupted prosody and distorted articulation. In other cases, the dysphasia is more severe. However it is much easier to differentiate the dysphasic and dyspraxic elements of the patient's problem, even to the extent of differentiating the dysphasic phonological impairment (literal paraphasia) from the errors of articulatory dyspraxia. Because the patient's language ability is higher than in previous groups and articulation is not so severely impaired, the extensive use of articulation drills in treatment becomes a possibility and the prognosis for improved speech is usually very good.

(f) Mild disorder

Some of these patients present with an apparently isolated articulatory dyspraxia though closer scrutiny may reveal the presence of a mild or even moderate degree of dysphasia, either concurrent or present in the early stages of recovery. However the patient's articulatory difficulty is the most obvious element of his disorder. His speech may also contain dysphasic phonological errors (literal paraphasias). The prognosis is usually very good although perfect speech probably should not be expected even at this high level. (Phonetic and phonological analysis of the speech of such patients might reveal a very interesting picture of the nature of speech impairment in dyspraxia and dysphasia.)

(g) Minimal disorder

These patients have barely perceptible problems to the layman, though they are often very aware of the difference between their speech before and after cerebral trauma. They require great concentration to speak well and speech may be slow and dysfluent. There may be an accompanying dysphasia but it may be minimal. Such patients can often do a great deal to help themselves in treatment. They will probably have very high expectations of returning to normal and, with luck and hard work, all such patients should eventually pass as normal speakers. However, some will continue to be aware of being slower in speech and language skills than previously, especially when under stress or feeling tired.

Treatment

The following examples of treatment of patients with both dysphasia and articulatory dyspraxia are drawn from several years of clinical practice. They are representative only in as much as they typify the patients encountered by this author. With so much variability in both the dysphasic and dyspraxic components of such communication disorders, as well as in the personalities and educational levels of the patients, it is impossible to be truly representative. However it is hoped that the following examples, mentioned briefly in *Aphasia Therapy*, Code and Muller, 1983, will give some useful guidelines on the selection of appropriate treatment techniques.

The emphasis in the following sections is inevitably on the treatment of the dyspraxia present. It is assumed that the reader is fully aware of the need to treat any concurrent dysphasia and is familiar with the relevant therapeutic procedures which will not be covered here except where they overlap with treatment of the dyspraxia.

(a) Treatment of gross disorder

In those patients with the severest form of dyspraxia the duration of the problem is highly relevant. Many patients may be grossly disordered in the acute and very early stages of recovery from cerebral trauma. Time and diagnostic therapy will tell whether they are likely to make rapid improvement or not. The patient who is chronically grossly disordered has a far different prognosis; and though a period of diagnostic therapy is indicated, its emphasis is usually different, concentrating on exploring alternative methods of communication rather than on recovery of speech, when the limitations of the latter have been categorically revealed. Wertz et al are at pains to make this distinction and discuss in detail both the general and specific needs of severely apraxic patients. (Their 'severe' category almost certainly incorporates both the 'gross' and 'very severe disorders' described in this volume.)

Where there is limb apraxia

Assessment and treatment of these severely impaired patients can be complicated by the presence of a severe degree of limb apraxia such that even pointing to command is affected. If such an ideomotor apraxia of the unparalysed arm exists it may well be appropriate to spend time working on volitional pointing with a view to helping the patient use a communication board. Once a patient can point consistently to command, it also makes cooperation with the comprehension section of standardized aphasia tests a great deal easier.

Sometimes it is easier to start with as few as two objects or pictures which are as visually, conceptually and phonetically different as possible, eg. a car and an apple. Careful explanation is needed so that the patient understands that he is just required to point in response to the clinician's stimulus. The latter can be a verbal request with or without a visual cue appropriate for the object, depending on the patient's verbal comprehension. At this stage the aim is to train the patient to point rather than to test his verbal comprehension. Sometimes it helps to guide the patient's hand in a pointing gesture whilst saying 'point to . . .' or 'show me . . .', and this may be repeated several times. Hopefully some progress will be made such that training can continue with the use of a communication board. Unfortunately as all clinicians will be aware, however well a patient performs with his board in clinical sessions, using it effectively for communication is another matter even when ward staff or relatives are very supportive. It is often disappointing to see how little useful carry-over there is into real communication situations in some cases; but it is certainly worth trying since some patients can and do transfer this skill.

Equally at risk from ideomotor apraxia of the unparalysed arm is the ability to use gesture to communicate. These grossly affected patients may have no spontaneous gesture at all and find it extremely difficult to imitate even the simplest gestures. Once again a few sessions are needed to establish whether the patient can utilize gesture at any level. The clinician must ascertain whether he can understand simple gestures, starting with one or two which are very easy to comprehend and easily imitated. Imitation of the selected gestures is the next step with the clinician 'moulding' the patient's hand if necessary. Production of the gesture to command or in response to a picture, object or written stimulus, or combination of these, comes next. The most difficult step is for the patient to use the gesture to communicate eg. either to answer a question or to describe a picture. If he shows the ability to learn gestures in this way, there is some hope that he may master a gestural system such as Makaton or Amerind. Even if complete mastery of a formal system is not possible, the patient may learn enough to enhance his communicative ability and may be encouraged to use natural signs more frequently and flexibly. However the presence of a severe limb apraxia often seriously limits the progress patients can make with gestural systems. Where limb apraxia is slight or absent, even if articulatory dyspraxia and dysphasia are severe, a gestural system such as Makaton or Amerind may help improve comprehension and expressive speech as well as providing a means of communication. Skelly's (1979) work is essential further reading. If the patient is unable to learn a gestural system but shows progress with a communication board, it is tempting to try a visual pictographic system, eg. Bliss symbolics, to extend communicative efficiency. However, as discussed in Chapter 4, little work has been reported using such systems with dysphasic and dyspraxic patients. Stella Bailey's case report is the exception and deserves careful study.

So far only alternative methods of communication have been considered and these are certainly most appropriate where the prognosis for recovery of speech and language is poor. However, all patients who are well enough to cooperate, deserve a trial period of work on oral speech production so that any patients with some prospect of recovering some speech are given the opportunity to show what they can do. (The same must also be said of work on language with those who are severely dysphasic.) It is important to note that patients who are grossly disordered in the very early stages may show rapid improvement and become progressively more able to cooperate with oral speech production tasks, whereas those with chronic long-term apraxia of speech are likely to show little or no ability to learn and carry over oral speech tasks.

Where there is oral apraxia

Once again non-verbal apraxia, in this case oral or bucco-facial apraxia, may be present and may make any work on articulation difficult if not impossible. However, as mentioned before, oral apraxia can exist in the presence of good articulatory ability though this is usually the case in Wernicke's rather than Broca's aphasics. It may be useful to work on facial gestures eg. smiling frowning, nodding and shaking the head, to reinforce these as a means of communication if the patient is able to cooperate.

Voluntary vocalisation may be absent in the very early stages of recovery and some time may have to be spent on eliciting voicing. This may be derived from coughing, grunting or laughing or other natural activities where vocalization does occur. Direct stimulation of the larynx by touch or massage with the patient feeling his own and the therapist's larynx may also be helpful. Once voluntary voicing is achieved, the aim is to prolong it then repeat it, reducing the amount of stimulation and facilitation required in stages as rapidly as the patient's successful production will permit. Once the patient is able to vocalize consistently, work on oral speech production may be started, utilizing a variety of techniques which will be described in the next section.

Where progress is minimal

If the patient is chronically grossly apraxic and aphasic the therapist has to accept, after a trial period of work on speech and language, that further progress is extremely unlikely. The clinician's time and energy must then be focused on exploring alternative means of communication as outlined here, and on helping both patient and relatives to accept the limits of progress. Any residual communicative ability such as drawing, if it is acceptable to both patient and family, needs to be encouraged.

It is important for both patient and relatives, even when the prognosis for recovery of speech and language is this limited, to see that as normal a life as possible is maintained. Alternative social outlets may be useful; if the patient wishes, participation in the general social activities of a stroke club such as outings or a weekly meeting, may be beneficial in providing moral support. Naturally, if he can maintain contact with previous non-verbal social outlets, so much the better. Outside contact and activities for the patient also mean that relatives get a break from the demands and frustrations of living and coping with someone so impaired in communicative ability. The relatives themselves may also benefit from attending a relatives' support group where the emphasis is on group counselling and where members help each other to cope with the changes in their lives. It is important that both patient and relatives are encouraged to look at those things in their lives which are still possible, concentrating on the patient's strengths rather than his disabilities – though this is much easier said than done. Finally it must be remembered that even if recovery of speech is impossible, some small degree of improvement in language skills (particularly comprehension) may occur over a period of time provided the patient has sufficient general language stimulation and is not allowed to become totally depressed and isolated.

Case study

T was a case who exemplified many of the problems to be found in grossly disordered patients. He was a comparatively young businessman, only 48 years old, who suffered a massive CVA leaving him hemiplegic, aphasic and apraxic. His family responsibilities included a wife and pre-school son.

Initially T was unable even to vocalize and could not communicate in any way at all, which gave rise to immense frustration. All attempts at direct work on speeech in the first few weeks simply intensified this frustration and led to very limited progress indeed. Unfortunately he was only receiving once-weekly treatment which was far from ideal (but nevertheless not unusual at that time). After several weeks' work on speech, during which time language was also assessed and treated, he was able to produce /ɑ/ and /m/ with much facilitation. The techniques used included direct manipulation of the articulators; mirror work which was quickly abandoned as of no benefit because his only response to it was to inspect his teeth and tidy his hair; derivation using a yawn to elicit /ɑ/ and a spontaneous utterance 'humph' to elicit /m/; and articulatory diagrams to help remind him and his wife of what we were trying to achieve. The amount of effort on everyone's part to elicit just these two sounds was enormous, and attempts to sequence them met with little success. Teaching of new sounds was thwarted by a strong tendency to perseverate.

Understandably, only a portion of each speech therapy session could be spent on such demanding work; but the patient's wife was asked to try the same techniques at home for a short time every day. Since she sat in on every session, she knew what was required and what to expect. The remainder of each session was spent exploring and stimulating T's language skills. Reading and writing were severely limited by aphasia; and his comprehension of speech was very variable. He also had a severe ideomotor apraxia of the left (unparalysed) arm and was initially unable to imitate gestures, though as time went on he began spontaneously to utilize one or two gestures, eg. rubbing thumb and fingers together was his sign for money. Even his ability to indicate 'yes' and 'no' was inconsistent. However, he did have some residual drawing ability so it was decided to try to teach him a simple pictographic communication system (Cameron, 1976). He was beginning to show some ability in this area but plainly resented working on alternative means of communication even though speech work was intensely frustrating. Both he and his wife appeared to be unable, at that stage, to accept the very limited speech prognosis.

In fact, T suffered a further CVA and died before any satisfactory conclusions could be reached about the pictographic system being tried. In retrospect, had his health and the time available allowed, further efforts could have been made to improve his gestural skills in addition to encouraging drawing and use of the pictographic system. The latter would have served a useful purpose in enabling T to assemble messages at his leisure, whereas the former would have been valuable for immediate communication. In fact encouragement of total communication was an aim of treatment. More time spent on counselling, particularly with his wife, would have been of immense value.

This case illustrates not only the very limited progress which many grossly disordered patients make but also the virtual impossibility of achieving worthwhile results on a once-weekly treatment basis. However it is impossible to predict if more progress would have been made in some aspect of communication with more intensive help. Another major drawback of once-weekly therapy was that counselling time was severely restricted. Ideally, far more time would have been devoted to this. Finally, the importance of the patient's state of health is underlined here. T was recovering from his CVA but his health was obviously precarious. We may well have found that he was physically unable to cope with the demands of intensive therapy, had it been available to him.

Summary of treatment aims: gross disorders

- Explore all communicative channels: trial treatment with communication board.
- Explore oral speech capability: trial treatment.
- Explore gestural ability: trial treatment.
- Explore visual symbolic skill (drawing and writing) with trial treatment if appropriate.
- Work on any dysphasia present.
- Counsel patient, relatives and ward staff as appropriate.

(b) Treatment of very severe disorder

Some patients who appear grossly affected in the first few days after CVA will rapidly progress to this stage. Others present at this stage and will also show rapid improvement in the early stages to a higher level. However, many patients will present with this level of communication difficulty three months or more post onset. Once again the prognosis depends, amongst other things, on the time post onset that this stage is reached.

Some such patients will have severe oral apraxia, severe limb apraxia and severe dysphasia in addition to severe articulatory dyspraxia. As mentioned previously, many find work on oral speech extremely difficult and initially frustrating. It is therefore tempting for therapists to concentrate their efforts on language work appropriate to the degree of dysphasia present, and on exploring alternative means of communication such as facial gesture, natural limb gesture and signing (as with grossly affected patients).

In spite of the effort involved, however, it is well worth spending part of each therapy session in diagnostic treatment working directly on speech, as this can pay dividends eventually. Where there is careful explanation of the articulatory problems and the value of the chosen therapeutic techniques, most patients are very willing to cooperate in spite of the difficulties. Many such patients have poor proprioceptive abilities and thus need a great deal of sensory stimulation and feedback to compensate for this deficit. Some, particularly those with severe dysphasia, will also have inadequate auditory monitoring.

Getting speech going

There are a variety of techniques for eliciting speech at this level, some of which have been described in detail in the previous chapter. Obviously if patients are able to imitate, there is no need for recourse to more intrusive methods. However, most patients at this level of severity will need all the help they can get. When simple imitation is not possible such techniques as phonetic derivation are needed; and where these are found too difficult, PNF and other direct manipulation of the articulators. The use of ice to reinforce position sense has been described in Chapter 5. Sometimes a therapist will move back and forth between these techniques, stimulating more directly as required and then 'standing back' when possible to encourage more imitative responses. Luria (1970) suggests the use of automatic activities as a means of phonetic derivation such that a yawn may be used to elicit /ɑ/, a hum to elicit /m/, singing 'la la' to elicit /l/ etc. Wertz et al describe methods of deriving a variety of sounds, eg. /f/ from gently biting the lower lip, /p/ from damming with the lips and /t/ from clicking the tongue as in derision (tut tut). Voice may be derived from humming, grunting, animal sounds or coughing; and vowels by combining voicing with the clinician's manipulation of tongue, jaw and lips. Wertz suggests combining phonetic derivation with phonetic placement as described by Van Riper and Irwin (1958). First the patient is given a description of how a movement or sound is to be made. Then associations (like derivations) are made; graphs, models and other visual aids are used; and the patient's articulators may be manipulated. In this way the patient is taught manner distinctions (/s/ versus /t/), manner and place distinctions (/t/ versus /f/), voice distinction (/p/ versus /b/) and oral/nasal distinction (/ɑ/ versus /m/). Keeping the patient informed of what the exercises are meant to achieve can be a useful motivator and ensure full cooperation. Such a very direct approach to articulation work is most likely to succeed where the patient is predominantly dyspraxic with only a mild or moderate degree of dysphasia and thus has good comprehension of what is required and a sufficient vocabulary to cooperate. The more severe the degree of accompanying dysphasia, the slower progress is likely to be and obviously the less effective the outcome for overall communicative ability.

Feedback of performance can be provided directly by the therapist or by a tape recorder or Language Master. The use of a mirror is not always successful, as mentioned before, and video taping may be discouraging rather than encouraging though this very much depends on the individual concerned and on the way it is used. The most effective stimulus for the patient is to have the therapist providing an audio-visual model, sitting where her face can be clearly seen and uttering the target slowly and clearly ie. providing a 'slow motion speech' model. This technique leads into the 'listen and watch me' approach described by Rosenbek in his 'eight-step continuum' and becomes more valuable as the patient improves. A useful way of reinforcing articulation work is by using articulatory diagrams (articulograms) as described in Chapter 5. A further technique described by Wertz et al is the use of strong rhythm to elicit speech. However they do not go so far as to recommend the Melodic Intonation Therapy programme for dyspraxic patients. It seems likely that the latter is much more appropriate where the patient is predominantly aphasic rather than apraxic, and as we have seen they did not find it helpful with patients who were predominantly dyspraxic.

Some patients treated in the ways described above will make steady progress, particularly where treatment can be both intensive and extensive and where home practice is encouraged. However, there is no doubt that the effort involved is enormous and the patient needs to be both fit enough and highly motivated to cope. In addition the gains may be limited so that the end result is no more than a small spoken vocabulary which would need to be supplemented if possible by gesture, writing and drawing, ie. total communication. Only the patient can decide if the effort involved is worth while (clinicians are naturally biased to think so!). Such therapy is very demanding on the clinician since a great deal of expertise is required regarding the different techniques and also great flexibility in their application is most likely to achieve good results.

Case study

Mrs M was a 47-year-old housewife who suffered a CVA which left her severely dysphasic, dyspraxic and hemiplegic with a mild degree of ideomotor apraxia of her left (unparalysed) hand. Her regular treatment continued for a period of two years though, as with other cases described, this was only on a once-weekly basis with her husband carrying out homework with her between sessions. Once again this was far from satisfactory but an unavoidable arrangement unfortunately all too familiar to many therapists. Much work was carried out on her dysphasia, with work on speech comprehension and written language, throughout her treatment. In the early stages much time was spent on articulation, first on voicing and then on isolated consonants and vowels. Most of the techniques already described were used, namely manipulation of the articulators, phonetic derivation, icing, 'listen and watch me' and the use of articulatory diagrams (see the examples in Chapter 5). Mirror-work was not found to be helpful. As soon as she was able, work began on simple CV and VC combinations introducing real words as early as possible and gradually building up the number of phonemes available and the complexity of the syllables used. The patient found speech work extremely demanding so it was generally carried out in short bursts, interspersed with language work which she found much easier. Over a period, it became obvious that speech would remain limited and it was decided to teach her some Amerind signs to broaden her communicative ability. She mastered the basic signs quickly with encouragement from her husband, and began to use some spontaneous signs too. In retrospect, the use of gesture should have been introduced much earlier in her treatment programme. After two years of therapy everyone concerned felt she had obtained the maximum benefit from individual speech therapy though further slight improvement in her overall communicative ability was not impossible, provided that she practised the skills she had acquired regularly in everyday communication situations. Both she and her husband accepted the termination of regular treatment sessions; but to ensure that she had some social stimulation, arrangements were made for her to attend a supportive speech therapy group.

Summary of treatment aims: very severe disorder

- Explore all communicative channels.
- Work on oral speech production using a variety of facilitation techniques.
- Work on gesture if necessary to complement oral speech and reduce frustration.
- Work on dysphasia present and the use of written language, again to complement oral speech.
- Counsel patient, relatives and staff.

(c) Treatment of severe disorder

The patients in the next three categories ie. severe, moderate and mild-moderate are probably similar to those grouped together by Wertz et al as moderately apraxic, at least in so far as their dyspraxia is concerned.

Useful techniques

Once again the patient who presents at this level very early post CVA may show rapid improvement to a milder form, but those who function at this level three or more months post onset are liable to progress more slowly and maybe not as far. Some of the techniques already described may also be useful at this level, albeit only as temporary facilitators or props. Patients at this level can generally imitate some speech so that recourse to techniques such as icing, phonetic placement and phonetic derivation is less frequently required. Similarly the need for alternative means of communication is less pressing and the patient himself is less likely to want to use such alternatives since he and his relatives naturally still regard speech as the main mode of communication.

These patients generally benefit from a 'listen and watch me' approach along the lines of Rosenbek's eight-step continuum (described in Chapter 3). The use of 'slow motion speech' models by the clinician, leading to the reauditorization techniques described by Schuell, is particularly appropriate. Visual reinforcement of the auditory pattern using articulatory diagrams is again very helpful. It is generally very much easier at this level to build up a selection of CV, VC and CVC combinations by these methods and to move steadily on to more complex combinations. These will be real words as far as possible, and used in appropriate linguistic contexts so that the patient becomes able to produce meaningful words early on in treatment. The degree of dysphasia present will obviously affect just how far and how fast such progress can be made.

Case study

Mrs L was a 60-year-old who had a CVA a year before starting regular speech therapy. She was rated as severely disordered at a year post onset (on assessment she was classified as a severe Schuell group 3), but having had no speech therapy up to that point, treatment was started with some optimism. She presented with some speech but her writing was severely impaired. She responded well to language stimulation techniques and her treatment programme included work in all language modalities. However, expressive speech was often unintelligible because of her severe dyspraxia. A combination of techniques was used to deal with the latter, emphasis being placed on 'listen and watch me' and reauditorization.

The results were particularly encouraging in view of the time lapse since her CVA. Only occasionally were more intrusive facilitatory techniques required. All speech work was reinforced with the written form. Homework was sent back to the old people's home where she lived, where staff were very willing to help. Communication with the staff at the home was by note and telephone. Undoubtedly a home visit would have been of even greater value. Nonetheless, Mrs L made good progress over the nine months she attended for therapy and this was reflected in reports from the staff at the home who were better able to understand her and found her much more willing to communicate than previously.

Summary of treatment aims: severe disorder

- Work on any dysphasia present.
- Use 'listen and watch me' and reauditorization to work on speech, reverting to more intrusive techniques only if necessary.
- Use articulatory drills including prosodic approach if the patient can cope.
- Counsel patient and relatives or staff as before.

(d) Treatment of moderate disorder

Since patients at this level present talking, it is generally easier to assess the comparative severity of the dyspraxic and dysphasic elements of their disorder and in some respects easier to plan appropriate treatment, dovetailing language and articulation work.

Useful techniques

The patient generally has more language available, making the use of articulatory and prosodic drills (eg. contrastive stress drills) more appropriate to treatment than in previous cases. Techniques of phonetic placement and derivation are rarely if ever needed. As before, a patient who presents at this level early after CVA is likely to make rapid progress whereas one who functions at this level after several months will take longer to effect improvement.

The most appropriate techniques at this level revolve around reauditorization, with a slow motion speech model by the clinician as a primary stimulus to imitation, and the use of articulatory drills. Since the patient can generally imitate, if very inaccurately at times, the use of a tape recorder or Language Master in therapy can be very helpful. Some patients are able to tape and monitor their own performance, which is a useful way of learning to self-correct.

Where the patient is also dysphasic, speech work can be integrated with language work to the benefit of both. Rosenbek's eight-step continuum is particularly appropriate at this level. The patient is usually able to make good use of auditory cues so that the 'watch me' element in stimulation can soon be dropped, progress to simple imitation being more rapid. Phonetic contrast drills (where manner, place, voice and resonance contrasts are emphasized) and contrastive stress drills (as described in Chapter 5) can be carried out much more effectively at this level, as can other techniques using prosody as an aid to fluency.

Those patients who are rather more dyspraxic than they are dysphasic will particularly benefit from the kind of articulatory drills described by Wertz et al. In this approach, imitation of phonetic contrasts is seen as the 'cornerstone' of treatment. At stage 1 the target eg. /s/, is imitated in a variety of phonetic settings such as 'saw', 'say', 'sew'. Stage 2 involves contrasting the target with another consonant, eg. drilling pairs of words such as 'see-tea' or 'sigh-tie'. Stage 3 focuses on harder contrasts and moves from monosyllabic to polysyllabic settings, also altering rhythm and stress as the patient progresses. Fawcus et al (1983) also describe methods of eliciting and drilling such minimal pairs. Such techniques as phonetic contrast drills and contrastive stress drills are generally appropriate to more moderately impaired patients rather than those with a severe disorder who may find the exercises rather too difficult. The word-retrieval techniques described by Fawcus et al (1983) are very useful where dysphasia and articulatory dyspraxia combine to render speech nonfluent. Such techniques as using forced alteratives, or 'wh' questions have been described in more detail in Chapter 5. Both Fawcus and Wertz recommend the use of what is effectively syllable-timing and stress-patterning to help with fluent production of polysyllabic words, phrases and sentences (see Chapter 5). Wertz favours the use of illustrative gestures to enhance stress patterns and reinforce contrastive stress drills, as previously described, whereas Fawcus et al simply refer to the patient beating out the required rhythm. The latter authors also suggest, as an exercise, the use of set intonation patterns as in reading aloud football results, announcing train arrivals, gale warnings and news broadcasts etc.

Case study

JF was a young graduate who suffered a CVA following cardiac surgery when he was 24 years old. Initially he was severely dysphasic, dyspraxic and hemiplegic, but by the time the author encountered him 2 years post onset, he was moderately dysphasic and dyspraxic and still hemiplegic. He lived alone and appeared to cope to his own satisfaction with the requirements of daily living. He had already had a considerable amount of speech therapy in the early stages of recovery, whilst living in a different town, and was able to communicate adequately, if very slowly and telegrammatically and with what appeared to be a foreign accent. He had decided that he wanted to improve his speech further so, with some reservations, he was taken on for a further course of treatment.

Because of the length of time since his CVA and the amount of previous therapy (and in additioin the fact that only one or two sessions of therapy a week would be possible) treatment aims were limited to a few restricted goals. It was decided to work towards improving certain aspects of written and spoken language and to attempt to improve articulatory accuracy and agility. Phonetic analysis of his speech revealed a strong tendency to palatalize alveolar and palato-alveolar sounds, thus giving rise to the 'foreign' sounding accent, so articulation drills concentrated on /ʃ/, /tʃ/, and /s/. At one stage an oscilloscope was used as a visual aid, in an attempt to reinforce the difference between his production and the target and this did seem to help in the short term. He was intelligent and cooperative and able to work alone to some extent with carefully prepared tape-recorded exercises aimed at improving auditory and written language skills whilst increasing awareness of phonetic sequencing. Writing to dictation from tapes became a regular piece of homework at one stage.

Whilst treatment continued, JF made and maintained progress but it required considerable effort and commitment on his part. When regular speech therapy sessions ended he lacked the motivation to keep up the standard he had reached during therapy. He is an example of the type of case who would benefit from extremely long-term follow-up with occasional 'top up' periods of speech therapy, if such could be arranged. One therapeutic approach which might have been very beneficial in this case, is the use of assignments to help with carry-over of gains made in treatment sessions into communication situations in everyday life. Ideally, such assignments should be routine with all higher-level patients who can cope with them. In addition role play could well have played a valuable part in bridging the gap between treatment sessions and real life.

The limit of JF's progress was not surprising in view of the time elapsed since his CVA and the amount of progress he had already made in the 2 years before we saw him. However he carried on leading his own life, learned to drive an invalid car and moved once again, appearing to have come to terms with the level of functioning which he had attained.

Summary of treatment aims: moderate disorder

- Work on dysphasia as appropriate.
- Combine language and articulation work whenever possible.
- Use 'slow motion speech' and reauditorization as appropriate.
- Utilize articulation drills and prosodic aids to fluency.
- Reinforce articulatory patterns and sequences through all modalities.
- Use role play and assignments to help carry-over achievements in clinical sessions to everyday communication situations.
- Counsel patient with regard to possible return to employment or alternative lifestyle where appropriate.
- Encourage all aspects of communication including writing, as speech cannot necessarily be relied on in every situation.

(e) Treatment of mild to moderate disorder

Patients at this level are usually able to communicate quite effectively using speech though this is often slow and effortful and has obvious distortions and disturbed prosody. The degree of dysphasia present may be very variable but it is generally very much easier to assess both dysphasic and dyspraxic elements of the problem and to carry out linguistic and phonetic analysis of the patient's speech, when an adequate speech sample can be obtained. Such analysis is not only an essential prerequisite to treatment at this level, but is also of academic interest since it often reveals the mixture of phonetic and phonological problems which tend to overlap in dysphasic dyspraxic patients. As Rosenbek points out, future research needs to link such phonetic findings with physiologic measures to give us a real insight into the processes involved in apraxia of speech. Individuals who are found to function at this level in the early stages of recovery generally have quite a good prognosis, though they are still likely to experience communication problems to some degree even after extensive treatment. There is more likelihood of patients in this group wishing to return to work, though only a percentage of them will be able to, and many of these may well need to return to a modified form of employment. For the majority, early retirement is the most likely option.

Useful techniques

The use of role play and assignments for encouraging carry-over from clinical sessions into functional communication situations becomes increasingly important at this and higher levels, since the patient is likely to have higher aspirations along with a better prognosis. Because of this he is likely to find himself in more demanding communication situations than someone more severely impaired who may be comparatively sheltered. The use of assignments can also help the clinician to evaluate the effectiveness of her therapy in real terms. In addition the true extent of the patient's difficulties is likely to be revealed. It is vital that both patient and therapist work together towards realistic goals and that sights are not set too high. Feedback and discussion after assignments is most important.

Techniques found most beneficial at this level are reauditorization (particularly where dysphasia is a problem) and articulatory drills of various types, as described in Chapter 5. The patient generally moves quite quickly from CVC combinations to di- and polysyllabic words and then to consonant clusters. Where there is also dysphasia and associated phonological confusion (literal paraphasia) reflected in speech and writing (eg. the patient not only says 'tup' for 'cup' but writes it too), the use of auditory discrimination training (both inter- and intra-personal) is indicated. Inter-personal auditory discrimination exercises are those where the therapist gives the patient a choice of 2, 3 or 4 words, pictures or objects with similar sounding names and asks him to choose the one she says. Intra-personal discrimination is the patient's ability to recognize his own errors: initially this may be recognizing his own tape-recorded production errors. The therapist helps by drawing his attention to appropriate phonetic contrasts by saying, eg. 'Do you mean sea or tea!' The patient relies heavily on the therapist to draw his attention to his errors. It is obvious from the above example that patients who are purely dyspraxic do not need this kind of therapy. They are only too well aware of their own errors. However, those who are also dysphasic (and those who are fluent dysphasics with many phonological speech errors, but who do not have articulatory dyspraxia) often need a great deal of help with such tasks. Wertz also suggests that it is debatable whether such auditory discrimination training is appropriate when the patient is purely dyspraxic, though improvement in self monitoring is always useful. Thus, where dyspraxia is the primary problem the emphasis is on articulatory drills and *not* on auditory discrimination.

Case study

Mr D suffered a CVA at the age of 61 and was moderately dysphasic with mild articulatory dyspraxia. His speech was also affected by dysphasic phonological impairment (literal paraphasia) and this combination rendered his speech quite unintelligible at times. Writing was comparatively well preserved and even early on in treatment he would attempt, sometimes successfully, to write a word he could not say. Treatment involved considerable work on language in all modalities, with a great deal of reauditorization and the use of slow-motion speech models, all reinforced in writing. Work on auditory discrimination and sequencing of phonemes was also emphasized.

At a later stage of recovery, sequences of pictures which told a story were frequently used for all aspects of language work. (A particularly useful series was one by L A Hill, aimed at older children, which incorporated picture sequences and written passages about the same material. This proved acceptable material from many points of view, including content.) Comprehension work involved selecting one appropriate picture out of eight, to verbal command or written command. Mr D was asked to try to describe individual pictures in his own words and also to tell the story. His attempts were used to make structured sentences for practice orally, and later for use as dictated sentences. He was also asked to attempt written description of the pictures, initially on a sentence-completion basis but gradually allowing him more scope for his own production. The written passage was used for practice in reading aloud and for reading comprehension. Last but not least, articulatory and phonological errors were picked up by the therapist as they occurred; and some time in each session was spent on auditory discrimination and on articulation using the polysyllabic words and consonant blends which had caused most difficulty. This rather broadly based strategy was deemed appropriate once again because therapy was limited to an hour once a week, which was far from ideal. In addition, Mr D found it hard to accept help from his wife so that scope for homework was limited to what he could achieve by himself.

After 18 months' treatment, during which he made slow but steady improvement, he was able to communicate quite well in a clinical situation, using speech supplemented by writing. There was, however, no question of him returning to work as a local government officer and he took early retirement. He appeared to be content to do this and to concentrate on his hobbies. He was fortunate in having no associated hemiplegia.

Summary of treatment aims: mild/moderate disorder

- Work on any dysphasia present as appropriate.
- Use reauditorization particularly where the patient is moderately dysphasic.
- Use articulatory drills extensively. Prosodic drills are particularly appropriate.
- Reinforce speech work with writing where possible and appropriate, and encourage all aspects of communication.
- Utilize assignments both to gain insight into carry-over from treatment and to lead the patient into real communication situations.
- Counsel patient and relatives, especially with regard to whether return to work is possible or desirable.

(f) Treatment of mild disorder

The mild and minimal categories described here are equivalent to the mildly apraxic patients described by Wertz et al.

Patients who present at this level are fortunate in that the prognosis is normally very good, even if speech does not eventually sound entirely as it did prior to the cerebral trauma. Once again the prognosis varies with time post onset. If the patient has mild or no dysphasia the outlook is very good for effective communication to be established quickly. Articulatory dyspraxia may be the most obvious problem or even the only problem the patient has. However, many patients have a degree of dysphasia at some stage in their recovery and this may not have resolved rapidly.

Useful techniques

As before, if there is dysphasia present then it must be included in treatment plans. At this level the extensive use of intensive articulatory drills of increasing complexity is entirely appropriate. Wertz describes how contrastive stress drills can be expanded and extended at this level. If the patient is primarily dysphasic with mild dyspraxia, obviously the emphasis in treatment will have to be altered accordingly.

Patients who are primarily mildly dyspraxic have a very good prospect of returning to their previous employment though even at this level some modifications may be needed depending on what that employment was. In any occupation where public speaking or a great deal of verbal communication is involved, the patient may well find that his speech deteriorates under stress and that he cannot function effectively at the same level as before. The use of assignments and counselling is particularly important to help resolve these issues in the most satisfactory way.

In addition to working hard on articulatory drills the patient needs to learn to live within his speech limitations and to take time to self monitor and self-correct. Wertz points out that there is a danger at this level: because the patient appears so normal, both he and his relatives and employers may expect too much. The sequalae of even slight brain damage can lead to increased fatiguability, and allowance must be made for the effects of this in everyday life.

Case Study

Mr B suffered a mild CVA at the age of 75 and presented as being rather dysfluent. Assessment revealed that his dysfluency was due both to a mild degree of dysphasia (mainly word-finding difficulty), and to mild articulatory dyspraxia superimposed on dysphasic phonological impairment. He improved rapidly following his CVA, but his speech remained somewhat dysfluent. Therapy concentrated on very high-level language work with much verbal description, picture description and reading aloud. Self-monitoring was encouraged. His articulation was adequate when he slowed his rate of speech so this approach was reinforced in preference to using articulatory drills. It can be argued that more use could have been made of high-level articulatory drills; but once again this patient was only receiving once-weekly treatment, and he lived alone, so that conditions were not ideal for practising and benefitting from such drills. In addition he felt happy with the methods being used since 'going slowly' was an easier goal to achieve at 75.

Summary of treatment aims: mild disorder

- Treat any dysphasia present.
- Use high-level articulatory drills, extending this into reading aloud and spontaneous speech. Work on prosodic features.
- Encourage self-monitoring.
- Use appropriate role play and assignments.
- Counsel, where appropriate, on use of social outlets and return to work with a realistic work load.

(g) Treatment of minimal disorder

These patients naturally, have the best prognosis of all. If they function at this level post trauma they have obviously escaped lightly and may improve so rapidly and completely that speech therapy is never required. For those who improve less rapidly, speech may be slow and dysfluent for some time and the patient may have to concentrate particularly hard in order to speak well. Where there is little or no dysphasia the outlook for returning to normal communication is excellent.

Useful techniques

Depending on his age and educational level, the patient can do a great deal to help himself, even to the extent of being encouraged to make up his own drills based on examples provided by the therapist. Such patients can, if motivated, carry out extensive work themselves using a tape recorder. Reading aloud, descriptions of pictures, events, news items or TV programmes can all be utilized. The clinician can recommend the highest level of articulatory drills with much emphasis on consonant clusters, polysyllabic words and long and complex sentences. Even tongue twisters can be used at this level and when performed successfully, are a great boost to morale. The need for role play and assignments depends very much on the patient's level of confidence and ability to monitor himself and gauge the pressures of the communication setting. (Some people can pace themselves much better than others and have a more realistic approach to difficult situations.)

Case study

Mrs FS, a 28-year-old school teacher, suffered a CVA which initially caused moderate dysphasia and mild articulatory dyspraxia, both of which improved very rapidly. Because of her dysphasia, high-level work on all language modalities was carried out and articulation work was dovetailed into this. Though the latter commenced at the level of CVC monosyllables, the patient rapidly progressed to consonant blends and polysyllabic words. She was encouraged to draw up her own lists of words for practice and used a tape recorder at home to monitor her articulation drills and reading aloud. When she was discharged from therapy six months after her CVA she had no noticeable problems in communication. However, she herself was aware that she was somewhat slower in speech and needed to concentrate harder on what she wanted to say. The question of her return to work was complicated by her underlying medical condition, but on the basis of her speech alone she felt confident that she could have coped once again in the classroom.

Summary of treatment aims: minimal disorder

- Treat any dysphasia present.
- Encourage self sufficiency in communication.
- Utilize the highest level of articulation drills and pay attention to prosodic features too.
- Use role play and assignments to get carry-over and improve confidence if necessary.
- Counsel as appropriate concerning return to work.

CHAPTER 7
TERMINATING TREATMENT

Treatment regimes/74
Terminating treatment/75
Summary and conclusions/76

CHAPTER 7
TERMINATING
TREATMENT

Treatment regimes

In an ideal world, the dyspraxic patient would have access to as much treatment as he needed to make optimum progress. In the real world this rarely occurs, whether in private practice or in the National Health Service. It seems very unfair that the opportunity for 'intensive' speech therapy is not equally available to all dyspraxic patients. Those who live in big cities near to teaching hospitals or other centres of excellence are most likely to be offered such intensive treatment. The rest must, it seems, be satisfied with once or twice-weekly sessions. Only a small percentage of speech therapists in Britain undertake private work with adult patients so that there is little opportunity at present for private therapy to supplement, or substitute for, NHS treatment. Areas with a limited speech therapy service are also unlikely to have a high proportion of private practitioners, with the result that in some parts of the country provision is grossly inadequate. Since intensive therapy cannot yet be provided for all, a common substitute is to make treatment *extensive* relying on the help of relatives or volunteers to work with the patient between clinic sessions. For some dyspraxic patients, particularly those with severe or moderate apraxia and a degree of dysphasia, a combination of both intensive and extensive treatment is required if they are to make satisfactory progress, that 'long gruelling process' described by Rosenbek. The very severely and grossly impaired patients, who are both dysphasic and dyspraxic, need an initial intensive burst of diagnostic treatment followed by extensive support, particularly if they are being encouraged to use alternative means of communication.

In these very severe cases the relatives may also need support for a considerable time and this is where long-term stroke clubs and relatives' support groups have a particular role to play. Such groups need not be run by a qualified speech therapist though it is always desirable to have the expertise of the clinician readily available. Such groups should be run under the supervision of qualified staff wherever possible.

Another alternative is the open-ended aphasic group such as that run at City University Stroke Group in London, where qualified staff and students work with the patients in a group and individually over a very long period of time. The group is not merely a supportive one but aims to provide a socially and therapeutically stimulating environment where long-term progress can continue to be made. A very wide range of dysphasic patients is treated at the City University Stroke Group, including those with varying degrees of articulatory dyspraxia. Further details of this group can be found in *Working with Dysphasics* (Fawcus et al, 1983).

It is much easier to define the limits of treatment for patients who are only mildly affected, and to think in terms of a course of treatment lasting a specified period of time and covering discrete speech, or speech and language, problems. Most of the patients described in Chapter 6, with the exception of Mr B and Mrs FS, were more profoundly affected than this. As a whole, these cases were not untypical in that their opportunities for intensive therapy were severely restricted. They also covered a very wide range of severity and combination of dysphasia and dyspraxia, so that no one treatment regime was suitable for all patients. Frequently a set regime could not be followed through rigorously with a particular patient, either because of infrequent treatment sessions or because of lack of resources (including specialist training) or both. Such patients were selected for inclusion in Chapter 6 because they represent the types of cases frequently encountered in clinics and illustrate the need for a flexible approach in dealing with their problems. They are not show cases, portraying ideal clinical practice, but demonstrate what frequently happens. As clinicians we must continue to strive and hope to improve our own levels of specialized training and other resources in our clinics, to the benefit of our patients.

Terminating treatment

The whole question of terminating treatment is thus partly dictated by the level of service available in the area where the patient lives and the ease of access to that service. Where there is heavy pressure on resources, decisions may have to be made to limit the amount of treatment available. Therapists are obliged to treat less frequently than they would wish, or to offer intensive treatment but for a strictly limited period. Many therapists using the former approach find it extremely hard to discharge their apraxic patients since there is always the feeling that just a little more progress might be made, or that the patient will regress when treatment stops. It is very helpful if criteria can be laid down at the start of treatment and adhered to: in other words, realistic long and short-term aims need to be clearly defined on the basis of a thorough assessment at the outset of treatment. When those aims are fulfilled it is much easier to feel justified in discharging the patient from regular speech therapy. It is also a help to the patient if he is aware of the aims of his treatment in broad terms so that he knows what *he* is aiming for. Similarly, a patient whose performance has reached a plateau and who shows no further signs of improvement on reassessment can be said to have gained maximum benefit from regular speech therapy, at least for the time being. The offer of follow-up appointments and further therapy in the future (if it seems appropriate) can often help to smooth the transition at the end of regular treatment, for all parties concerned. Finally the use of supportive stroke groups or clubs can be of great value in maintaining levels of speech performance and especially morale.

As we tighten up our assessment procedures and become more rigorous in evaluating the effectiveness of treatment, it may become a little easier to make decisions about terminating therapy. It should certainly help the clinician to concentrate on those methods which produce the best results and to abandon those long-favoured techniques which are subsequently found, an objective analysis, to produce minimal benefit.

The potential gains from speech therapy for any individual depend on so many factors, all of which have to be considered when evaluating the prognosis. There will always be some patients who confound our early predictions for one reason or another. Factors such as general health, personality, mental state, support from relatives and home environment all have a bearing on the final outcome of therapy, even if the precise cause and effects are sometimes difficult to identify. Aetiology, size of lesion, localisation, severity and time post onset are known to be specific factors affecting the prognosis in aphasia and very likely in apraxia too.

With regard to the patient who is primarily dyspraxic, with little or no dysphasia, Wertz et al show that improvements can be expected even when the apraxia is severe. However, such patients tend to be exceptional; and in the average caseload the majority tend also to be dysphasic. In such cases, the prognosis is bound to be affected by the degree of dysphasia. In this volume we have concentrated on the types of cases most commonly seen in our hospital clinics (ie. those who are both dysphasic and dyspraxic), rather than on the more exceptional patients with an isolated articulatory dyspraxia. All comments about prognosis and treatment, therefore, have been made with this context in mind.

SUMMARY AND CONCLUSIONS

An attempt has been made in this volume to draw together briefly and concisely what is currently known about the assessment and treatment of articulatory dyspraxia; and this has been specifically applied to the patient who is both dyspraxic and dysphasic. Progress in investigating the phenomenon of apraxia of speech has been very rapid in recent years. Almost as soon as we have grasped and applied one set of principles, new ideas emerge and new facts are discovered which cause us to modify our thoughts on this disorder and its treatment. A good example of the way such developments alter how we perceive our patients' problems is the now common distinction made between phonetic and phonological disorders – a distinction which is central to the approach to assessment and treatment of articulatory dyspraxia presented here. Clinicians are finding such a distinction very useful in practice; yet even as we utilize such 'new knowledge' in our treatment, phoneticians and linguists are modifying the rules! An excellent discussion of this very issue can be found by Harris and Cottam, and Hawkins, in *BJDC* (Volume 20, Number 1, 1985), and by Hewlett, Grunwell and Milroy again in separate papers in *BJDC* (Volume 20, Number 2, 1985).

Most of the treatment techniques described in this book have been popular for a considerable time, partly because they have been found to be effective clinically. The author does not claim to be expert in all the techniques described, but only to have had some clinical experience of most of them, a position which is not uncommon among clinicians. For this reason, references have been given throughout the text to the work of those who have been, or are emerging as, experts in the field of treatment of apraxia of speech. It is not yet known whether all the treatment techniques described will stand up to rigorous clinical trials of their efficacy. However, the assessment and treatment procedures covered here will provide a useful starting point for those clinicians new to working with dyspraxics. For those more experienced in this field, it is hoped that the Bibliography will provide fresh food for thought.

APPENDIX I
HUSKINS NON-VERBAL APRAXIA SCREENING TEST

Instructions for use

Materials

Paper and pencils, picture stimulus cards (*see Fig 3*), 6 match boxes and at least 8 matches.

Procedure

(i) The patient sits opposite the clinician. Both should have good light.

(ii) The clinician explains the purpose of the test. It is not a test of verbal comprehension but of the ability to copy oral and limb gestures and to make two and three-dimensional models.

(iii) The clinician asks the patient to do exactly what she says and does. (eg. 'Can you put out your tongue . . . (slight pause) . . . like this (demonstrates)?' The instructions may be repeated.

(iv) For the construction subtest, the three-dimensional designs are carried out first. The clinician builds a model using three match boxes on the table in front of the patient. She then gives him the three other match boxes and invites him to copy her model. For the drawing item, the pictures are presented one at a time and the patient is asked to copy them, using pencil and paper. The matchstick designs are also presented one at a time by the clinician; and the patient is given the appropriate number of matchsticks to copy each design. Further details can be found in Chapter 2.

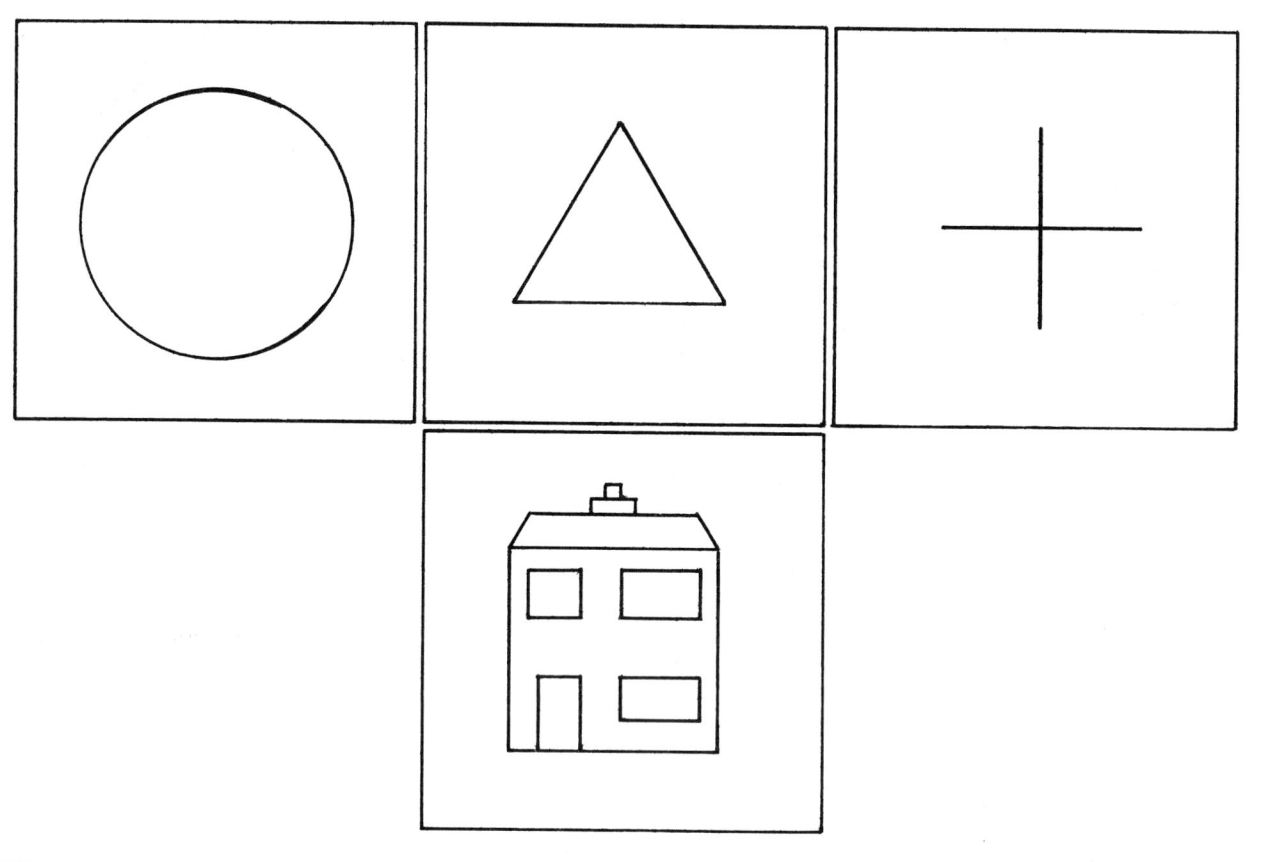

Figure 3. Stimulus pictures for constructional praxis subtest.

Figure 4. Example of normal performance on constructional praxis subtest.

(Using right and left hands alternately.)

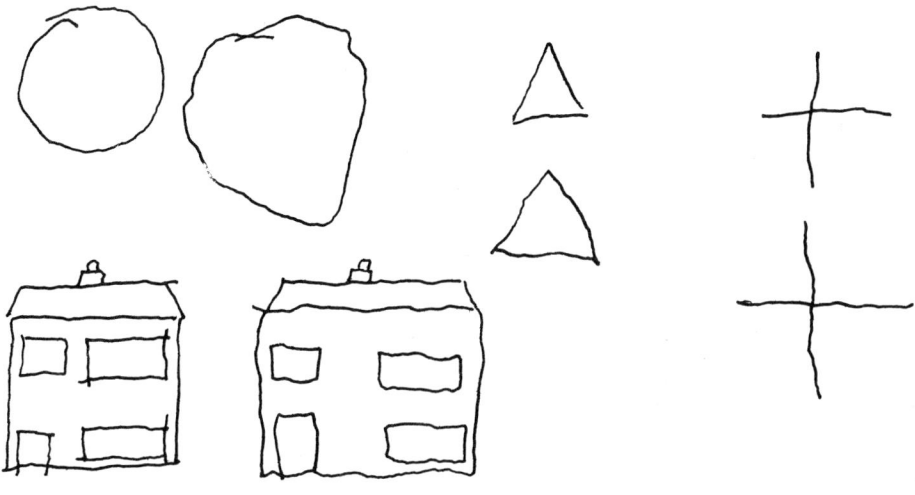

Patient's signature:

Figure 5. Two examples of abnormal performance in constructional praxis subtest.

PATIENT I

Scores:
circle – 2
triangle – 1
cross – 1
house – 0
Total – 4

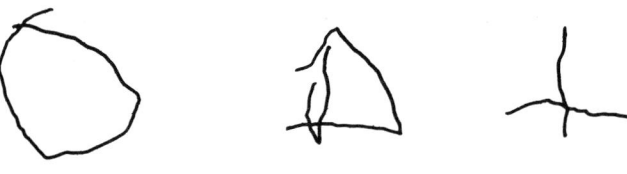

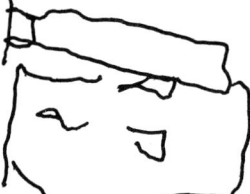

Patient's attempted signature:

PATIENT II

Scores:
circle – 2
triangle – 2
cross – 2
house – 0
Total – 6

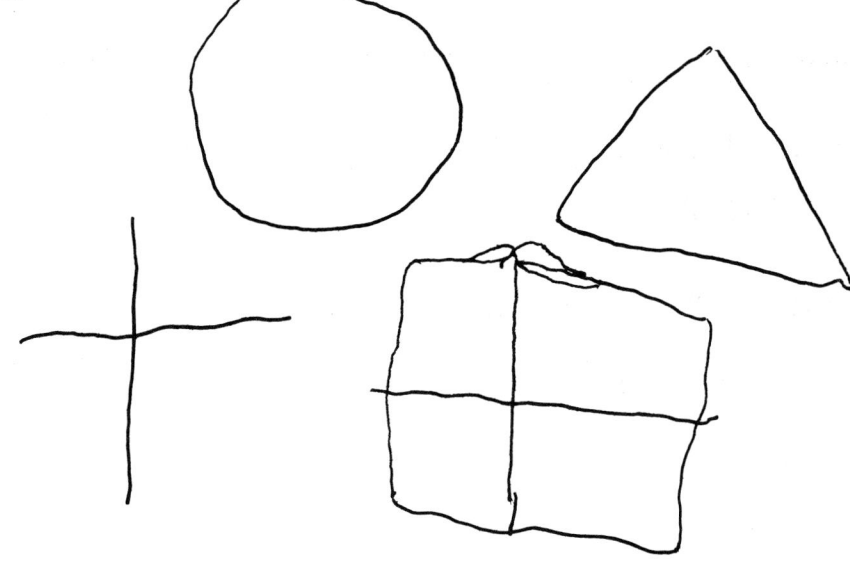

Patient's attempted signature

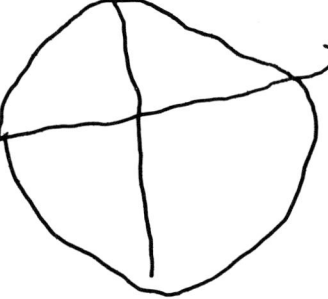

Huskins non-verbal apraxia screening test.

Name: Age:

Address: Sex:

Diagnosis: Occupation

Other assessments: Date:

ORAL PRAXIS	SCORE	COMMENT	IDEOMOTOR PRAXIS	SCORE	COMMENT
protruding tongue smiling looking glum swallowing licking lips whistling kissing blow out match smoke cigarette clicking tongue			make a fist thumbs up wave goodbye say/ʃ/ point way out salute victory V comb hair light match seal letter		
SCORE TOTAL:			SCORE TOTAL:		

CONSTRUCTIONAL PRAXIS   SCORE TOTAL:

3D: bridge   train   step

Drawing: circle   traingle   cross   house

Matchsticks: triangle   cross   square

Spontaneous writing:

Appendix II
DIAGNOSTIC CHECK LISTS

Instructions for use

The creation of these check lists is described in some detail in Chapter 2, as are the criteria for their use and the type of scoring systems which are appropriate. Where possible a full-scale analysis of the patient's speech is preferable: these check lists are seen as a screening procedure for busy clinicians.

General points

(Please read then proceed with caution!)

(i) Only to be used on adult patients with analyzable speech.

(ii) To be used in conjunction with other formal assessment procedures and test batteries and with information regarding the patient's medical and neurological status.

(iii) Used in this way the check lists may confirm or clarify a diagnosis which has already been tentatively made.

(iv) A tape-recorded sample of spontaneous speech is highly desirable (between 5 and 15 minutes in length, depending on the patient's rate of speech).

(v) The items in the check lists are not equally weighted nor are they intended to be.

(vi) The features listed in each check list are the most common factors representative of each condition. However, the presence of any one feature is not necessarily diagnostic of that condition. The more errors on any one list, and the higher the rating given, the more certain the diagnosis. The context of the errors is important as is the overall error pattern.

Rating Scale:	Averaged Scores:
0 = Feature Absent	0-0.5 = Negligible
1 = Minimal	0.5-1.5 = Minimal
2 = Mild	1.5-2.5 = Mild
3 = Moderate	2.5-3.5 = Moderate
4 = Severe	3.5-4.5 = Severe
5 = Very Severe	4.5-5 = Very Severe

Example

The following is an example of the results one might expect when using the check lists with a typical dyspraxic dysphasic patient with a right hemiplegia and right facial weakness. The individual check list scores can be found in the table on page 83; and calculation of the average severity rating (ASR) is included.

PATIENT'S PROFILE

Number of Features:	ASR:
Dysarthria – 6	0.7 (Minimal)
Dysphasia – 10	2.7 (Moderate)
Dyspraxia – 10	3.6 (Severe)

Individual check list scores

CHECK LIST 1 (Dysarthria)		CHECK LIST 2 (Dysphasia)		CHECK LIST 3 (Dyspraxia)	
Item	Rating	Item	Rating	Item	Rating
1	1	1	2	1	4
2	1	2	2	2	4
3	1	3	4	3	5
4	1	4	4	4	4
5	0	5	3	5	3
6	1	6	2	6	3
7	0	7	2	7	3
8	0	8	3	8	4
9	0	9	3	9	3
10	2	10	2	10	3
Total	7	Total	27	Total	36

To calculate:

$$ASR = \frac{Total}{10}$$
$$= \frac{7}{10}$$
$$ASR = 0.7$$
$$= Minimal$$

$$ASR = \frac{Total}{10}$$
$$= \frac{27}{10}$$
$$ASR = 2.7$$
$$= Moderate$$

$$ASR = \frac{Total}{10}$$
$$= \frac{36}{10}$$
$$ASR = 3.6$$
$$= Severe$$

Diagnostic check lists: dysarthria/dysphasia/ dyspraxia

Name: Age: Sex:
Address: Occupation:

Medical diagnosis: **Date:**

Additional handicaps:

Other assessments: **Date:**

Speech diagnosis: **Date:**

Patient's profile: **Date:**

Number of Features:	**Average Severity Rating:**
Dysarthria	A S R
Dysphasia	A S R
Dyspraxia	A S R

Comments

Signed:

Check list 1: Dysarthric features

PATIENT'S NAME

	Features	Rating(0-5)
1	There is evidence of neuromuscular weakness of the speech musculature.	
2	Speech musculature has abnormal range and speed of movement.	
3	There are changes in muscle tone eg. spastic or flaccid.	
4	Drooling present.	
5	Feeding difficulties present (difficulty swallowing; choking; regurgitation).	
6	Errors of stress, rhythm and rate occur.	
7	Errors of loudness, intonation and voice quality occur.	
8	Errors of oral and nasal resonance occur.	
9	There are phonetic distortions of a consistently similar type.	
10	Articulation rate is abnormal.	

TOTAL FEATURES

TOTAL RATING

AVERAGE SEVERITY RATING (A S R)

Other comments

Signed:

Check list 2: Dysphasic features

PATIENT'S NAME:

	Features	Rating (0-5)
1	Syntactic errors present.	
2	Morphological errors present.	
3	Semantic errors present.	
4	Word-finding errors present.	
5	Phonological errors present. Phonemic selection and sequencing errors occur, eg. consonant substitutions, omissions, transpositions and insertions.	
6	Perseveration occurs at word level.	
7	Perseveration occurs at sound level (consonant harmony).	
8	Phonological errors reflected in writing.	
9	Linguistic errors reflected in all modalities.	
10	Auditory comprehension, discrimination and monitoring impaired.	

TOTAL FEATURES

TOTAL RATING

AVERAGE SEVERITY RATING (A S R)

Other comments

Signed:

Check list 3: Dyspraxic features

PATIENT'S NAME

	Features	Rating (0-5)
1	Groping for articulatory postures can be seen.	
2	Such groping can be heard (phonetic experimentation).	
3	Dysfluency at an articulatory level occurs.	
4	Speech generally slow and laboured in the absence of significant muscular weakness.	
5	Frequent repeats and attempts at self-correction.	
6	Variable phonetic errors occur, eg. weakening.	
7	Phonetic sequencing errors occur.	
8	Speech errors increase with articulatory complexity.	
9	Production of non-English sounds occurs.	
10	Production of non-English sequences occurs.	

TOTAL FEATURES

TOTAL RATING

AVERAGE SEVERITY RATING (A S R)

Other comments

Signed:

APPENDIX III
ARTICULATORY DIAGRAMS

These articulatory diagrams are modified from the ones drawn for the author by John Cameron (as described in Chapter 5). As far as possible the full range of English phonemes has been covered. Diphthongs have not been included since, if needed, they can be built up from other vowels. The lip positions for the vowels have been exaggerated, as has the degree of mouth opening, to give a clearer picture of the tongue position than could be seen in a photograph. Obviously it is impossible to indicate any allophonic or regional variation in such a simplified scheme. (In practice, this does not seem to matter since the diagrams are used at a point in therapy when the clinician is getting speech going, concentrating on the production of isolated sounds and simple sound combinations.) They are not appropriate at higher levels of ability when such subtleties might be important.

An attempt has been made to write the sound pictured using the English alphabet rather than phonetic symbols. This is so that patient and helpers have a chance of reading the sound appropriately; but even so, explanation is required for some items. The diagrams are arranged phonetically for ease of access by the clinician and in such a way that photocopies can be made and used as appropriate. A reduced size set of the diagrams is also provided, to increase the flexibility of the system.

Plosives

p

/p/

b

/b/

t

/t/

d

/d/

k

/k/

g

/g/

Fricatives

f

/f/

v

/v/

th

/θ/

TH

/ð/

s

/s/

z

/z/

Fricatives

sh

/ʃ/

zh

/ʒ/

Affricates

ch

/tʃ/

dg

/dʒ/

Fricative

h

/h/

Lateral glide

l

/l/

Glides

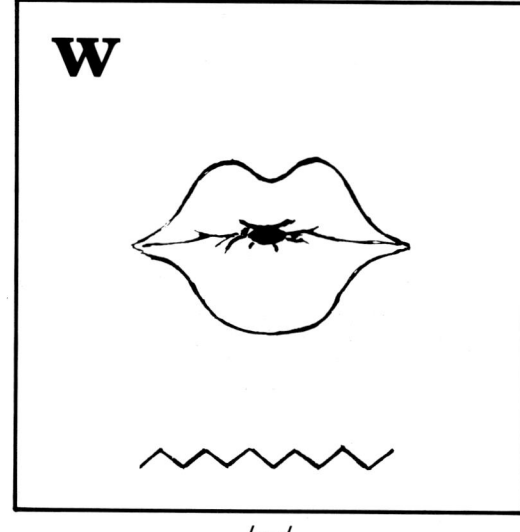

/w/

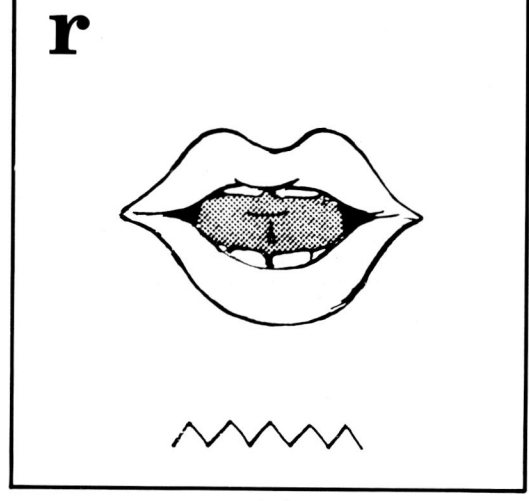

/r/

Glide

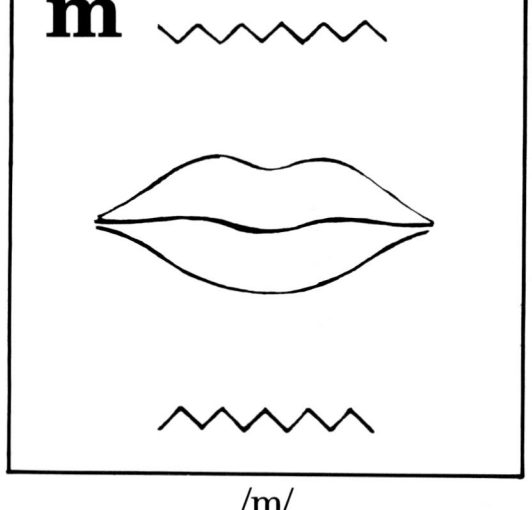

/j/

Nasal

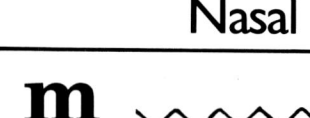

/m/

Nasals

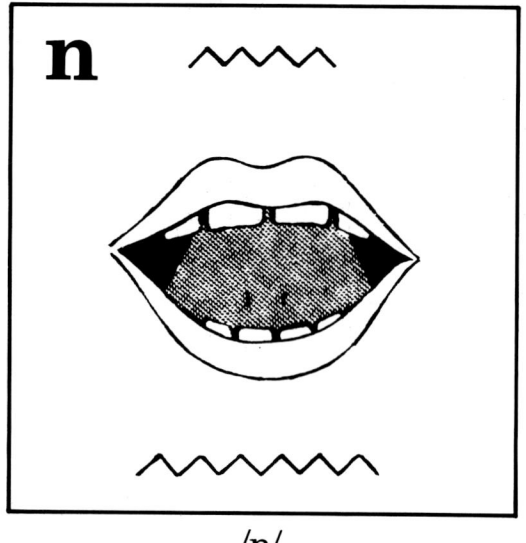

/n/

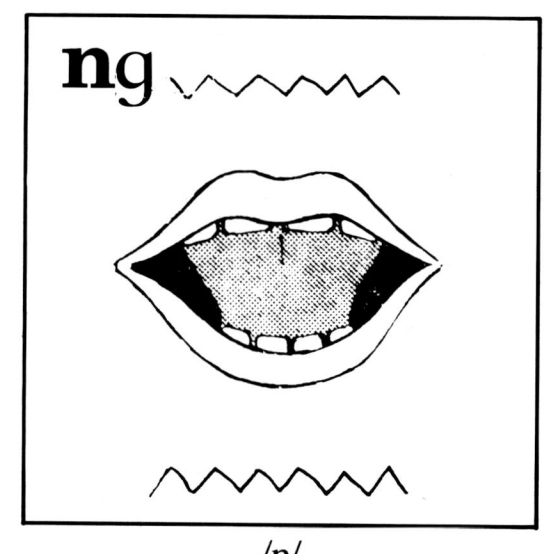

/ŋ/

92

Vowels

ee

/i/

i

/ɪ/

e

/e/

a

/æ/

ah

/ɑ/

o

/ɒ/

Vowels

oo

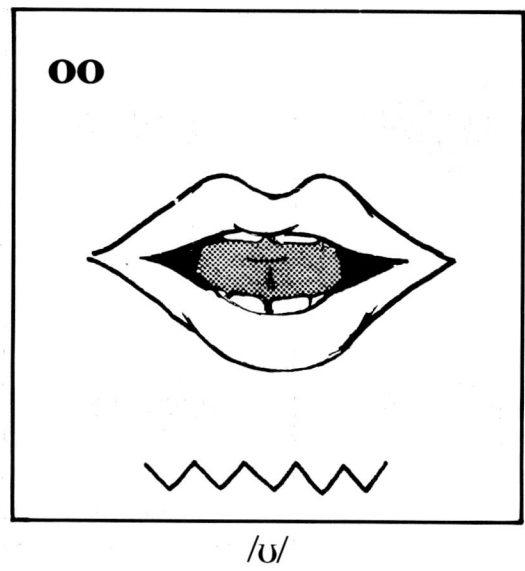

/ʊ/

or

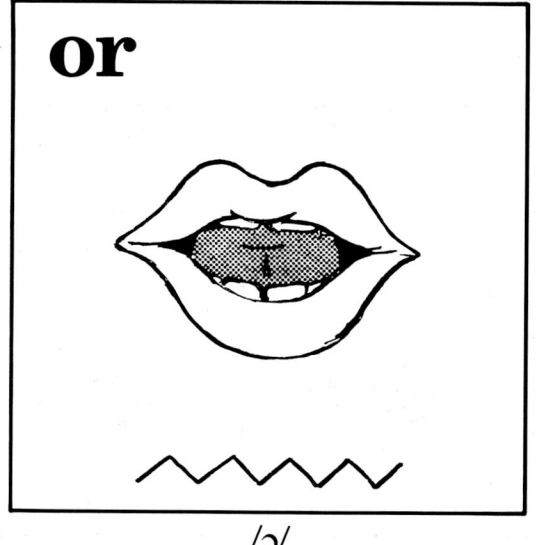

/ɔ/

oo

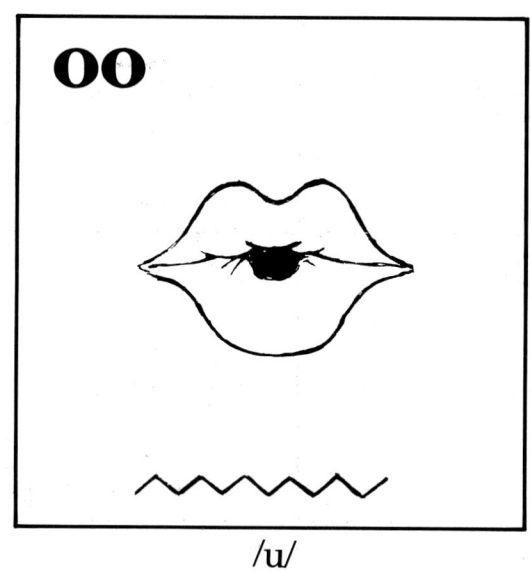

/u/

u

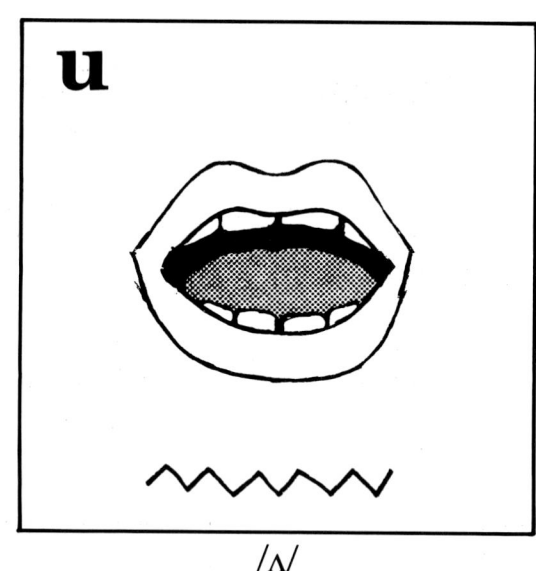

/ʌ/

ir

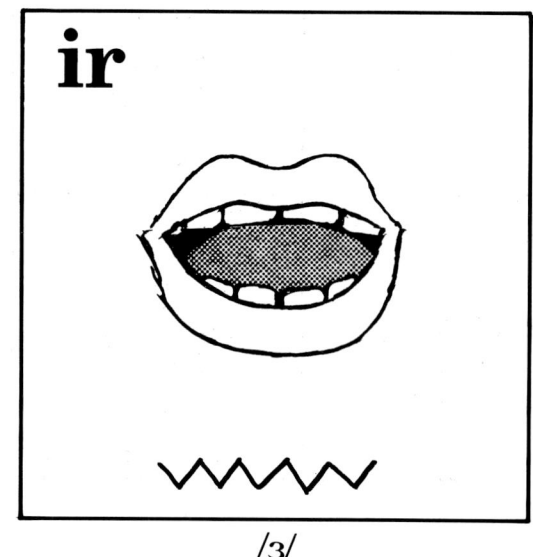

/ɜ/

a o e

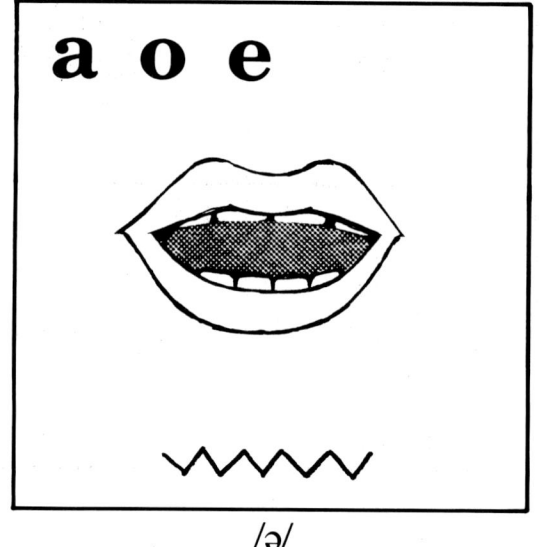

/ə/

Reduced size diagrams

p	**b**	**t**	**d**
k	**g**	**f**	**v**
th /θ/	**TH** /ð/	**s**	**z**
sh /ʃ/	**zh** /ʒ/	**ch** /tʃ/	**dg** /dʒ/
h	**l**	**w**	**r**
y /j/	**m**	**n**	**ng** /ŋ/

Reduced size diagrams

ee	i	e	a
/i/	/ɪ/	/e/	/æ/

ah	o	oo	or
/ɑ/	/ɒ/	/ʊ/	/ɔ/

oo	u	ir	a o e
/u/	/ʌ/	/ɜ/	/ə/

APPENDIX IV
PROSODIC AND ARTICULATORY DRILLS

The clinician should explain to the patient that they are to practise a word containing a particular target sound, in a particular position, using a question-and-answer format. The patient is given the answer that he must produce, so that he can concentrate on his articulation of the word when he answers the clinician's carefully structured questions. Sometimes these may be forced alternatives, where the required answer appears in the question. More difficult are straight questions: these can be structured to require a one-word answer if desired or made more difficult by requiring several words including the stressed target.

The following examples contain a variety of answer types. This type of exercise can be varied to drill sounds in a variety of positions in the stressed word. Wertz et al suggest five rules for the use of contrastive stress drills. Firstly, the drill must be constructed round one or a limited number of targets. Secondly, the target must be a sound that the patient can produce normally *sometimes*. Thirdly, word and total utterance length need to be controlled. Fourthly, the target sound must be placed appropriately in the word (final or medial sounds are often easier than word initial sounds). Finally, the other sounds required should be those which the patient can already produce easily. Bearing this in mind, the drills listed below are examples of the types which might be useful.

Examples of Contrastive Stress Drills

PLOSIVES:

1   Target: word initial /p/

Example 1

Clinician: Did he receive the letter?
Patient: He *posted* it.
Clinician: Did you receive the letter?
Patient: I *posted* it.

Example 2

Clinician: Did you drink beer?
Patient: I drank *pop*.
Clinician: Did you drink milk?
Patient: No, *pop*.

2   Target: word initial /b/

Example 1

Clinician: Did you sell the car?
Patient: I *bought* it.
Clinician: Did you steal the car?
Patient: No, I *bought* it.

Example 2

Clinician: Did you eat a sandwich?
Patient: I ate a *bun*.
Clinician: Did you eat an apple?
Patient: No, a *bun*.

3   Target: word initial /t/

Example 1

Clinician: Did you cut that?
Patient: I *tore* it.
Clinician: You broke it?
Patient: No, I *tore* it.

Example 2

Clinician: Would you like coffee?
Patient: I would like *tea*.
Clinician: Did you say coffee?
Patient: No, *tea*.

4   Target: word initial /d/

Example 1

Clinician: Did he swim in shallow water?
Patient: *Deep* water.

Clinician: Was it shallow?
Patient: No, *deep*!

Example 2

Clinician: Did the victim live?
Patient: He *died*.
Clinician: Did he recover?
Patient: No, he *died*!

5   Target: word initial /k/

Example 1

Clinician: Would you like bread or cake?
Patient: I would like *cake*.
Clinician: Did you say buns or cake?
Patient: *Cake*!

Example 2

Clinician: Is he brushing his hair?
Patient: No, *combing* it.

Clinician: Is he washing his hair?
Patient: He is *combing* his hair!

6   Target: word initial /g/

Example 1

Clinician: Is scrabble a sport or a game?
Patient: A *game*.
Clinician: Is Bridge a sport or a game?
Patient: A *game*.

Example 2

Clinician: Is he coming or going?
Patient: *Going*.
Clinician: Are you staying at home?
Patient: No, I'm *going*!

AFFRICATES:

1   Target: word initial /tʃ/

Example 1

Clinician: Will you saw the wood?
Patient: *Chop* it.

Clinician: Will you stack the wood?
Patient: No, *chop* it!

Example 2

Clinician: Is the dog on a rope?
Patient: He's on a *chain*.
Clinician: Is he on a lead?
Patient: No, *a chain*.

2   Target: word initial /dʒ/

Example 1

Clinician: Is the milk in the bottle?
Patient: In the *jug*.
Clinician: Is it in the saucepan or the jug?
Patient: The *jug*.

Example 2

Clinician: Will the man fall?
Patient: No, *jump*.
Clinician: Fall or jump?
Patient: *Jump*!

NASALS:

1   Target: word initial /m/

Example 1

Clinician: Did you buy that?
Patient: I *made* it.

Clinician: You found it?
Patient: No, I *made* it!

Example 2

Clinician: Was that your dad?
Patient: No, my *mum*.
Clinician: Did you say your aunt?
Patient: My *mum*!

2   Target: word initial /n/

Example 1

Clinician: Do you want to go later?
Patient: I want to go *now*.
Clinician: Do you want to go in half an hour?
Patient: No, *now*!

Example 2

Clinician: Did you hurt your elbow?
Patient: I hurt my *knee*.
Clinician: Did you hurt your ankle?
Patient: No, my *knee*!

FRICATIVES:

1   Target: word initial /f/

Example 1

Clinician: How many goals did they score?
Patient: *Four.*
Clinician: Did you say three?
Patient: No, *four*!

Example 2

Clinician: Will the weather be dull today?
Patient: *Fine.*
Clinician: Did you say cloudy?
Patient: No, *fine.*

2   Target: word initial /v/

Example 1

Clinician: Is he driving a car?
Patient: A *van.*
Clinician: Is he driving a bus?
Patient: No, a *van.*

Example 2

Clinician: Is the house on the hill or in the valley?
Patient: In the *valley.*
Clinician: Is it in the mountains?
Patient: No, in the *valley*!

3 Target: word initial /θ/

Example 1

Clinician: Have you hurt your finger?
Patient: No, my *thumb*.
Clinician: Your finger hurts?
Patient: My *thumb* hurts!

Example 2

Clinician: Are you going to the cinema?
Patient: To the *theatre*.
Clinician: Where are you going?
Patient: The *theatre*.

4 Target: word initial /ð/

Example 1

Clinician: Would you like these or those?
Patient: *Those*.
Clinician: Are you sure you wouldn't like these?
Patient: I'd like *those*!

Example 2

Clinician: Who broke the window?
Patient: *They* did.

Clinician: Wasn't it him?
Patient: No, *they* did it.

5   Target: word initial /s/

Example 1

Clinician: Did you hear the fight?
Patient: No, I *saw* it.

Clinician: You heard it?
Patient: I *saw* it!

Example 2

Clinician: Was he playing in the mud?
Patient: In the *sand*.
Clinician: Was he playing in the water?
Patient: No, the *sand*!

6   Target: word initial /z/

Example 1

Clinician: Did you go to the park?
Patient: No, the *zoo*.
Clinician: The Museum?
Patient: The *zoo*!

Example 2

Clinician: Do you button it up?
Patient: I *zip* it up.

Clinician: You tie it?
Patient: No, *zip* it!

7 Target: word initial /ʃ/

Example 1

Clinician: Did you buy a new hat?
Patient: New *shoes*.
Clinician: New socks?
Patient: No, *shoes!*

Example 2

Clinician: Will you keep all the apples?
Patient: I will *share* them.

Clinician: Will you sell them?
Patient: No, *share* them.

CONTINUANTS:

1 Target: word initial /w/

Example 1

Clinician: Is this made of plastic or wood?
Patient: *Wood.*
Clinician: Did you say metal?
Patient: No, *wood*!

Example 2

Clinician: Did you run or walk?
Patient: *Walk.*
Clinician: How should you cross the road?
Patient: *Walk.*

2 Target: word initial /l/

Example 1

Clinician: Was the book on a high shelf?
Patient: A *low* one.

Clinician: Did you say high?
Patient: No, *low.*

Example 2

Clinician: Is he sailing on a river?
Patient: No, a *lake.*
Clinician: Did you say a pond?
Patient: A *lake*!

3   Target: word initial /r/

Example 1

Clinician: Is her name Mary or Ruth?
Patient: Her name is *Ruth*.
Clinician: Did you say Ann?
Patient: No, *Ruth*!

Example 2

Clinician: Does the sun shine much in winter?
Patient: No, it *rains*.
Clinician: What happens when the clouds are black?
Patient: It *rains*!

4   Target: word initial /j/

Example 1

Clinician: Is a daffodil blue or yellow?
Patient: *Yellow*.
Clinician: Is your favourite colour blue?
Patient: No, *yellow*.

Example 2

Clinician: When you're tired do you smile?
Patient: I *yawn*.
Clinician: Do you groan?
Patient: No, I *yawn*.

NOTE

At a later stage, the stress pattern of the answer may be altered by restructuring the question, so that the target is no longer in a stressed position. This is helpful in developing a more normal stress contour.

BIBLIOGRAPHY

Bailey, S, Bliss Symbolics and Aphasia Therapy: a Case Study, in *Aphasia Therapy*, Eds Code, C, and Muller, D J, Edward Arnold, 1983.

Brain, L, *Speech Disorders, Aphasia, Apraxia, Agnosia*, 2nd edition, Butterworths, 1965.

Cameron, J A, A Proposal for Research in Visual Communication Systems for Aphasia and Related Conditions, unpublished MA thesis, Birmingham Polytechnic, 1976.

Code, C and Gaunt, C, Treating Severe Speech and Limb Apraxia in a case of Aphasia, Preprint, Leicester Polytechnic, 1986.

Coltheart, M, Aphasia Therapy Research: A Single-Case Study Approach, in *Aphasia Therapy*, Eds Code, C, and Muller, D J, Edward Arnold, 1983.

Critchley, M, *The Parietal Lobes*, Arnold, 1953.

Dabul, B, *Apraxia Battery for Adults*, C C Publications, Tigard, Oregon, 1979.

Dabul, B L and Bollier, B, Therapeutic Approaches to Apraxia, *Journal of Speech and Hearing Disorders*, 1976, 41, 268-276.

Darley, F L, Aronson, A E and Brown, J R, *Motor Speech Disorders*, 1st edition, W B Saunders, 1975.

Deal, J L and Florence, C L, Modification of the Eight-Step Continuum for Treatment of Apraxia of Speech in Adults, *Journal of Speech and Hearing Disorders*, 1978, 43, 89-95.

De Renzi, E Pieczuro, A and Vignolo, L, Oral apraxia and aphasia, Cortex 2, 1966.

Enderby, P and Hamilton, G, Communication Aid and Therapeutic Tool: A Report on the Clinical Trial Using Splink with Aphasic Patients, in *Aphasia Therapy*, Eds Code, C, and Muller, D J, Edward Arnold, 1983.

Fawcus, M, Robinson, M, Williams, J and Williams, R, *Working with Dysphasics*, Winslow Press, 1983.

Geschwind, N, *Disconnexion Syndromes in Animals and Man*, Brain, 1965.

Goodglass, H and Kaplan, E F, *The Assessment of Aphasia and Related Disorders*, Lea and Febiger, 1972.

Grunwell, P, *Clinical Phonology*, 1st edition, Croom Helm, 1982.

Grunwell, P, Comment on the Terms "Phonetics" and "Phonology" as applied in the Investigation of Speech Disorders, *British Journal of Disorders of Communication*, 1985, 20, 2.

Harris, J and Cottam, P, Phonetic features and Phonological features in Speech Assessment, *British Journal of Disorders of Communication*, 1985, 20, 1.

Head, H, *Aphasia and Kindred Disorders of Speech*, Hafner Publishing Co, 1963.

Heddel, F, *With a Little Help from the Chip*, British Broadcasting Corporation, 1985.

Hewlett, N, Phonological versus Phonetic Disorders: Some Suggested Modifications to the Current Use of the Distinction, *British Journal of Disorders of Communication,* 1985, 20, 2.

Hill, L A, *Picture Composition Book,* Longmans, 1960.

Hill, L A, *Teachers Guide to Picture Composition Book,* Longmans, 1960.

Huskins, S M, A study of Apraxia in Aphasic Adults, unpublished MSc thesis, University of London, 1973.

Huskins, S M, Treatment of Articulatory Apraxia in Aphasic Patients, in *Aphasia Therapy,* Eds Code, C, and Muller, D J, Edward Arnold, 1983.

Jenkins, J J, Jimenez-Pabon, E Shaw, R and Williams, J, *Schuell's Aphasia in Adults, Diagnosis, Prognosis and Treatment,* 2nd Edn, Harper and Row, New York, 1975.

Langley, J and Darvill, G, Procedures for Facilitating Improvements in Swallow, Mastication, Speech and Facial expression where these have been impaired by central or peripheral nerve damage, private publication, 1979.

Lesser, R, *Linguistic Investigations of Aphasia,* Edward Arnold, 1978.

Luria, A R, *Traumatic Aphasia,* Mouton, The Hague, 1970.

Luria, A R, *The Working Brain,* Penguin, 1973.

Milroy, L, Phonological Analysis and Speech Disorders: a Comment, *British Journal of Disorders of Communication,* 1985, 20, 2.

Philpott, A, Picturing Words, *College of Speech Therapists' Bulletin,* October, 1985.

Rosenbek, J C, Lemme, M L, Ahern, M B, Harris, E H and Wertz, R T, A Treatment for Apraxia of Speech in Adults, *Journal of Speech and Hearing Disorders,* 1973, 38, 462-472.

Rosenbek, J C, McNeil, M R and Aronson, A E, *Apraxia of Speech: Physiology, Acoustics, Linguistics, Management,* 1st edition, College Hill Press, San Diego, California, 1984.

Rowley, D T, Artificial Languages and Communication Aids in Aphasia Therapy, in *Aphasia Therapy,* Eds Code, C and Muller, D J, Edward Arnold, 1983.

Schuell, H, Jenkins, J and Jimenez-Pabon, E, *Aphasia in Adults,* Harper and Row, New York, 1964.

Skelly, M, *Amerind Gestural Code based on Universal American Indian Hand Talk,* Elsevier, New York, 1979.

Skelly, M, Schinsky, L, Smith, R W and Fust, R S, American Indian Sign (Amerind) as a Facilitation of Verbalisation for the Oral Verbal Apraxic, *Journal of Speech and Hearing Disorders,* 1974, 39, 445-456.

Sparks, R W, Holland, A L, Method: Melodic Intonation Therapy for Aphasia, *Journal of Speech and Hearing Disorders,* 1976, 41, 287-97.

Travis, A, Handbook of Speech Pathology, 1972.

Van Riper and Irwin, *Voice and Articulation,* Prentice Hall, Englewood Cliffs, 1958.

Vinken, P J and Bruyn, G W, Eds, *Handbook of Clinical Neurology,* volume 4, (Disorders of Speech, Perception and Symbolic Behaviour) 1970.

Wertz, R T, LaPointe, L L and Rosenbek, J C, Apraxia of Speech in Adults: the Disorder and its Management, Grune and Stratton, New York, 1984.

GLOSSARY

Aphemia. This is the term Broca used to describe what we would now call articulatory a/dyspraxia or apraxia of speech.

Apraxia of speech. An American term for a disorder of articulation in which there is obvious difficulty initiating utterances, articulatory inconsistency, effortful groping for the correct speech patterns, attempts at self correction, and disturbed prosody. It can occur in the absence of neuromuscular weakness or aphasia though it is more frequently found accompanying aphasia. The term is applied to all levels of severity, from the absence of speech to mild speech impairment.

Articulatory dyspraxia. This term is synonymous with the American term "apraxia of speech". However in England the term apraxia traditionally refers to absence of the praxic function and dyspraxia to disordered ability; hence the term articulatory dyspraxia is generally used when the patient has some speech which is disordered as described above. Articulatory apraxia refers to the total loss of the ability to speak in this context.

Isometric (static) resistance. A term used in PNF manipulation. The patient attempts to hold a position whilst the therapist applies pressure against the muscles involved.

Isotonic (moving) resistance. A term used in PNF manipulation. The patient moves muscles in opposition to pressure by the therapist.

Literal paraphasias. Also known as phonemic paraphasias (see below).

Modality. The mode of communication:
Auditory modality – that which is heard.
Graphic modality – that which is written.
Lexic modality – that which is read.
Oral modality – that which is spoken.

Phonemic paraphasias. These are dysphasic mispronunciations which are phonologically similar to the intended sounds. The errors obey the rules of English phonology. They involve such things as selection errors, perseveration and anticipation of sounds, omissions, insertions and metathesis.

Phonetic derivation. The use of automatic activities to facilitate the production of the desired sound (as described by Luria, Van Riper and others).

Phonetic errors. A variety of phonetic errors can be found in the speech of dyspraxic patients as described below.

(i) Idiosyncratic substitutions: Some dyspraxic patients produce sounds which are not normally found in the English phonetic inventory. When a patient has such favourite non-English sounds they are said to be idiosyncratic.

111

(ii) Phonetic experimentation: This describes the patient's attempts to produce the intended target sounds. This is sometimes done silently (but visibly) or audibly, when very quiet or 'weak' articulations may be heard as the patient tentatively tries out the sound. This phenomenon is also referred to as 'groping' towards the correct pronunciation.

(iii) Phonetic sequencing errors: These are sequencing errors produced by dyspraxic patients where consonant combinations materialise which do not obey the rules of English phonology.

(iv) Weakening of articulations: This often occurs in the process of phonetic experimentation.

Scan. This refers to the computer-enhanced imaging which is becoming routine in studying the brain and its pathology. A CT scan (computerised tomography) is based on conventional X-rays. Computer-enhanced images are produced using a sophisticated X-ray scanner such that great detail of internal structures can be seen and X-ray pictures of sections through the body or brain can be generated. Because of the danger from X-rays, the use of such scans has to be limited. NMR (nuclear magnetic resonance) or MRI (magnetic resonance imaging) scanners do not use X-rays but rely on the properties of atomic particles in response to a very strong magnetic field. Computer-enhanced images of very great clarity can be produced. This technique has the great advantage that it is quite safe so that repeated scans can be undertaken, thus building up the clearest pictures yet of internal organs such as the brain.

Abbreviations

BDAE – Boston Diagnostic Aphasia Examination.

CVA – Cerebro-vascular accident (eg stroke).

MTDDA – Minnesota Test for the Differential Diagnosis of Aphasia.

RTA – Road traffic accident.

PNF – Proprioceptive neuromuscular facilitation.

PICA – Porch Index of Communicative Ability.